Better Balance for Life

Banish the Fear of Falling
with Simple Activities Added to Your Everyday Routine

CAROL CLEMENTS

Foreword by Jon LaPook, MD

THE EXPERIMENT

NEW YORK

BETTER BALANCE FOR LIFE: *Banish the Fear of Falling with Simple Activities Added to Your Everyday Routine*
Copyright © 2018 by Carol Clements
Foreword © 2018 by Jonathan LaPook

The Experiment, LLC | 220 East 23rd Street, Suite 600 | New York, NY 10010-4658 | theexperimentpublishing.com

This book contains the opinions and ideas of its author. It is intended to provide helpful and informative material on the subjects addressed in the book. It is sold with the understanding that the author and publisher are not engaged in rendering medical, health, or any other kind of personal professional services in the book. The author and publisher specifically disclaim all responsibility for any liability, loss, or risk—personal or otherwise—that is incurred as a consequence, directly or indirectly, of the use and application of any of the contents of this book.

Many of the designations used by manufacturers and sellers to distinguish their products are claimed as trademarks. Where those designations appear in this book and The Experiment was aware of a trademark claim, the designations have been capitalized.

The Experiment's books are available at special discounts when purchased in bulk for premiums and sales promotions as well as for fund-raising or educational use. For details, contact us at info@theexperimentpublishing.com.

Library of Congress Cataloging-in-Publication Data

Names: Clements, Carol (Personal trainer) author.
Title: Better balance for life : banish the fear of falling with simple
   activities added to your everyday routine a 10-week plan / Carol Clements.
Description: New York : The Experiment, [2018] | Includes bibliographical
   references.
Identifiers: LCCN 2017026289 (print) | LCCN 2017030794 (ebook) | ISBN
   9781615194261 (ebook) | ISBN 9781615194155 (paperback)
Subjects: LCSH: Falls (Accidents) in old age--Prevention. | Exercise for
   older people.
Classification: LCC RC952.5 (ebook) | LCC RC952.5 .C54 2018 (print) | DDC
   617.10084/6--dc23
LC record available at https://lccn.loc.gov/2017026289

ISBN 978-1-61519-415-5
Ebook ISBN 978-1-61519-426-1

Cover and text design by Sarah Smith
Cover illustration by Amanda Sim
Illustrations by Amanda Sim
Author photograph by Ellis Michael Quinn

Manufactured in China

First printing November 2018
10 9 8 7 6 5 4 3 2 1

For Livia and Richard

Contents

Foreword
by Jon LaPook, MD

Carol Clements has turned her attention to a serious problem facing people as they age: the risk of falling and suffering a severe injury. The National Institute on Aging warns that more than one in three people 65 and older fall each year. Falls are the cause of most hip fractures, and many people who suffer hip fractures never get back to normal. The fear of falling can prevent you from staying active, and can lead to social isolation. Overcoming the fear can help you stay engaged and healthy.

Many things can increase the risk of falling— including medical problems; failing eyesight and hearing; unsafe footwear; alcohol consumption; subtle safety hazards, like loose rugs; sleep deprivation; and medications that cause side effects such as dizziness, sleepiness, or confusion.

There's no surefire way to improve balance, and serious falls sometimes happen despite best efforts to prevent them. But Carol Clements has reached into her decades of experience in exercise methods and movement arts to create a program that aims to improve balance by integrating exercise routines into the daily activities of life. She understands that there are countless excuses for avoiding the gym—so she removes the gym from the equation and replaces it with locations like the bedroom, kitchen, and bathroom. Her logic: you're there anyway, and with a little thought and practice, you can do exercises while drinking coffee, brushing your teeth, watching TV, rinsing dishes, talking on the phone, getting dressed, checking email, or even taking a shower.

Before following the *Better Balance for Life* blueprint, I recommend you check with your healthcare provider to make sure the suggestions in the book make sense for you. The National Institute on Aging provides advice on how to prevent falls and fractures; their website is nia.nih.gov/health/prevent-falls-and-fractures.

Here's to a healthy, happy, well-balanced life!

—Jon LaPook, MD
Chief Medical Correspondent, CBS News
Professor of Medicine, NYU Langone Health

Introduction

Are you afraid of falling? Do you find yourself holding on to something to keep your balance and feel safe? As my contemporaries and I entered our sixth decade, we baby boomers were all surprised—with many complaints—that we had to endure the aging process. In the past, Susan trotted down the stairs in the middle of the crowd, but now she steps to the side and holds the handrail. Rick was recently traveling in Europe and felt insecure walking on cobblestones. Anxiety struck when Bill found nothing to hold on to while navigating the stands at the baseball stadium. This is a generation like all generations. In youth, they took it for granted that they'd be active and agile forever. Now, they're losing confidence in their ability to do what formerly came naturally. They worry about losing their balance and falling.

As a personal trainer, yoga instructor, and dance and movement specialist for more than forty years, I've helped people become aware of their own physicality and to develop flexibility, coordination, and endurance so they feel healthy and energetic. We focus on increasing their muscle mass and density, so that these do not diminish with age. Together, my clients and I have peeled back layers of joint and muscle dysfunction so that their body mechanics and alignment support ease and mobility. This process takes time and commitment from my students and clients.

But not everyone can afford a personal trainer. And not everyone wants to put his or her time or money into that kind of individual assistance. Many don't like the idea of exercising. Some don't belong to a gym or attend scheduled classes.

That's why I wrote this book—to reinvigorate your balance and your physical well-being—without scheduled exercise sessions. In the next ten weeks, you will incorporate simple activities into your everyday life that will improve your agility and stability—and you won't even break a sweat!

Each week you add four simple activities to your daily routines, such as brushing your teeth, rinsing the dishes, putting on your socks, or sitting down to work at your computer. The challenges gradually increase in difficulty and as you progressively master each step in the program, you'll begin to notice that you've become more confident. When you can stand on one leg and button your shirt, you are ready to trust your ability to walk on uneven pavement.

You can stand up without holding on and have better balance for life and pleasure.

How to Lose Your Balance and How to Get It Back

You get it. The research shows that getting older is directly proportional to a loss of balance and the risk of falling. The potential reasons for problems with balance are many: medical conditions and side effects from prescription drugs, decreases in vision and reaction time, poor posture, muscle weakness in the hips and legs, gait pattern disorders, and the fear of falling itself. However, the main culprit for most of us can be summed up as: inactivity.

Activity is key. Activity will give you balance practice. Activity will give you strength. And that will give you confidence. The 10 Weeks of Daily Activities in this book are your foundation for a more active future. You can't do much about your advancing age, but you *can* intervene to improve balance, mobility, strength, and the self-assurance that arises from an appreciation of your own abilities. The goal of the ten weeks and its progression of activities is to practice balancing, build strength, and garner confidence to conquer the fear of falling.

Practice Balancing

Around the age of fifty-eight, when Jamie's cataracts got worse, the yellow and black painted stripes on the subway stairs presented an optical issue that her brain couldn't sort out. The result? She fell and sprained her ankle. Now she fears losing her balance, so she slows down and grips the handrail to feel secure.

Helping us stand balanced are our brain, nervous system, vision, inner ear, muscles, bones, and other body-orienting reflexes. As we age, our vision can become less reliable, which may lead to falls, but let's focus on the physical act of balancing. Jamie may or may not improve her vision, but she can improve her balance. She can practice balancing.

No matter what your age, if you're in a stable position, your body's balance system turns off. When you're sitting down, it's turned off. While you stand, it's switched on. As you age, you may spend more time sitting and less time standing. Herein lies the crux of the matter: Balance is a skill. It gets better with practice and deteriorates without it. When you limit your activities, you practice balancing less and therefore diminish your balancing skills. The solution is to stimulate your sense of balance by being in an unstable position while, of course, minimizing the risk of falling. You need to practice balancing, which is what we'll do in this book.

Build Strength

While walking in the mall, Eric found himself surrounded by quickly moving teenagers skimming past him. He didn't trust his ability to balance and needed something to hold on to while he sidestepped the commotion. This nervous moment brought the realization that he couldn't count on muscle power from his lower extremities to keep him from losing his balance.

Weakness in the lower limbs predicts a decline in balance. Strengthening his lower body will help Eric regain confidence in his balance.

You've got muscles! To increase your physical capabilities and improve your posture, activating muscles is essential. Throughout this book, you will engage your muscles by locating them in your own body. You will feel the sensation of the muscles engaging (contracting), and use that engagement for movement and stability.

Overcome the Fear of Falling

Here's a critical factor that contributes to the risk of falling—the *fear* of falling.

Many older adults who fall, and even those *who have never fallen*, express a fear of falling, and restrict their daily activities because of the fear. This sets up a vicious cycle that further reduces physical capability, promotes social isolation, and in turn, further increases the risk of falling.

This fear is damaging only if it interferes with physical and social mobility. Increased caution can be a good thing. There are times we all need to rein in our distracted rushing, slow down, be careful, and protect ourselves against falls. But activity-limiting worry can inhibit the very comings and goings and opportunities for balance practice that would help improve balance, muscle strength, and mobility.

On a snowy day, Rita, age fifty, was coming in for work at the hospital. The tile floor at the entrance was wet and mucky from foot traffic. You can imagine the rest of the story: Rita slipped and fractured her foot. Although the injury has long since healed, she continues to feel a lingering fear of falling. Rita admits that even when young she was afraid of walking on ice. These days, she doesn't go out as much, especially in the winter or at night. The fear hasn't lessened, even though she hasn't fallen again. She doesn't believe she'll ever feel entirely free of this fear.

Fear of falling is clearly identified as one of the most important and—here's the good news—*most modifiable* threats to autonomy in older individuals. You can enhance your physical activity and perform specific activities that reinforce confidence to decrease fear of falling.

Exercise intervention is an effective and proven way to decrease fear of falling. Following the training progression in this book produces benefits that will accumulate over time and show up in unexpected ways. Get ready for a rewarding return to mobility, confidence, and balance.

Reduce Your Risk Factors for Falling

You can't change your age but you can:

- Wear sensible and flexible-soled footwear
- Be careful about rugs and clutter in your home
- Light your living space better
- Improve your physical skills to counteract fear and avoidance behaviors in lifestyle activities.

Test Your Balance

How good *is* your balance and, more important, how do you react to balance challenges? Let's find out.

Stand behind a sturdy chair and place your hands lightly on the chair back for support. Place your feet right next to each other so they touch. Gradually let go of the chair and cross your arms over your chest. Slowly close one eye, and then the other, so that both eyes are closed.

Without using your sense of sight, observe what happens in your body from the inside. How comfortable are you with the wavering motion of instability? Where do you feel tension? Do you teeter to primarily one side or the other? Breathe and settle your weight if you can. Relax and experience the swaying. Stay with it for a while. Touch the chair back for support if you need to. Feel yourself balancing.

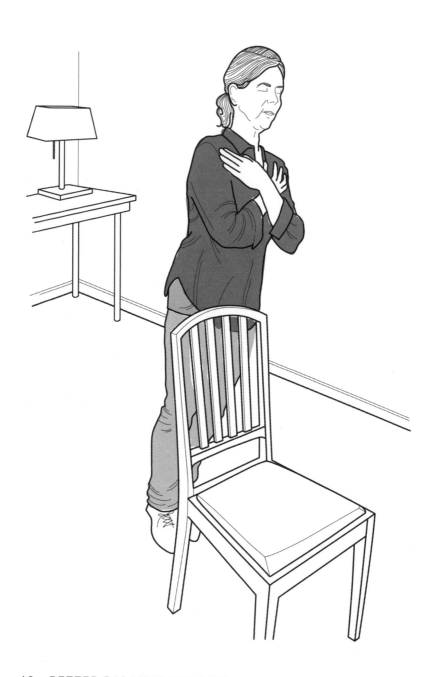

Five Principles of the Body in Balance

Here are five principles of the body in position to practice balancing. Before you begin the ten-week plan, get your bearings and experience lining up your posture. Let's start at the top with the head, neck, and shoulders, and go down the torso and hips to the feet.

1. The Head Floats like a Helium Balloon

Experiment with the relationship of your head to your neck. Push your face forward—in front of the rest of your body. Do you feel the compression behind your shortened neck? To decompress, tilt your chin toward your throat and glide your head backward behind your neck. Now the back of your neck is too flat and stiff! Release that tension.

Use the image of a helium balloon as the back of your head, behind your ears—not under your chin—so that the back of your neck lengthens and your head floats back and up instead of sinking forward. Imagine that your cheekbones are sliding backward, behind your shoulders. While your head floats up, your spine can fall like a string tied to the balloon. Your head can rotate more freely in this position and your posture has a head start for more ease in balancing.

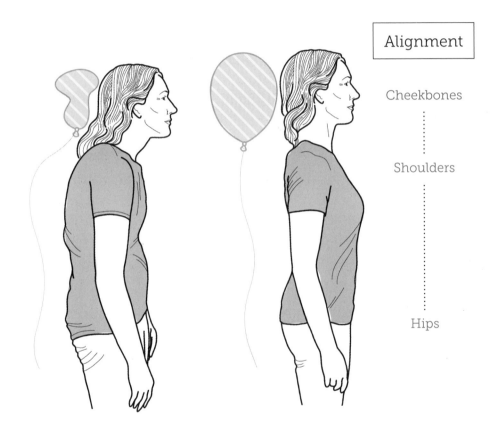

Alignment

Cheekbones

Shoulders

Hips

2. The Arms Belong to the Back

Have you noticed people who have rounded shoulders, causing their head to reach forward from their neck and deflate their helium balloon? This posture keeps muscles in their back from anchoring their shoulders down and along the sides of their back. If these muscles aren't activated, the arms become part of the neck and chest—which is not where they belong!

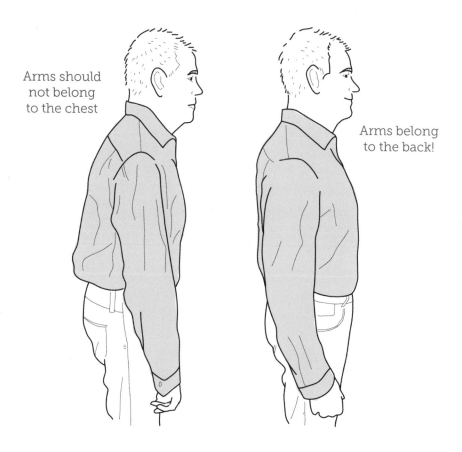

Arms should not belong to the chest

Arms belong to the back!

When the shoulders are not rounded, the upper spine can extend, allowing your shoulder blades to draw your arms into their shoulder sockets and slide down your back.

Years of rounding your upper back may have tightened your chest muscles. Before you can gain access to the muscles that draw your shoulders and arms into your back, you will need to open your chest. Take some time to experience a broader chest. For this you will need a large towel.

Roll the towel into a long cylinder and place it on the floor. Lie down with your spine stretching from head to tailbone upon the rolled towel. Place the soles of your feet on the floor with your knees bent, and relax your back. Let your shoulders drop so they fall behind your chest and towel onto the floor. You will feel a stretch across your chest to your armpits. Your shoulder blades will fall on either side of the rolled towel toward the floor. Now your arms have fallen away from your chest to their rightful place. They now belong to your back.

Raise your arms straight up to the ceiling and turn your thumbs outward. Now, keeping your arms straight, lower your arms directly out to the side to make a T at chest level. Once your arms are resting on the floor, relax your thumbs, leaving your palms up.

Breathe in to fill your lungs all the way above your collarbones and allow the top of your chest to expand.

Your upper spine will naturally lengthen with the inhalation. Relax your back and neck as you breathe. Don't tense your rib cage as a response to breathing fully or force your chest as a response to its stretching.

Your heavy shoulders and arms fall wide as you breathe in—from the bottom of your belly to the top of your chest.

When you exhale, empty the air in reverse order, breathing out starting from the top of your chest and completing the exhale from the bottom of your belly.

Start all over again and fill yourself with air from the bottom to the top. Empty from the top to the bottom. Continue to breathe until you feel less of a stretch sensation across your upper chest.

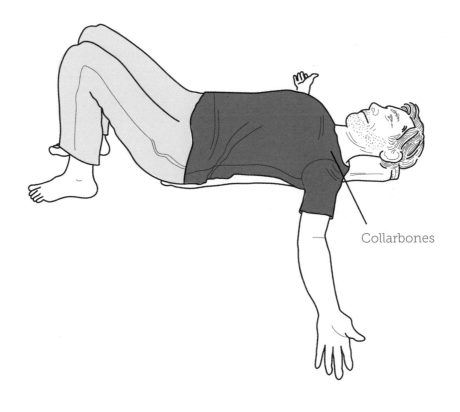

Collarbones

When you stand up, notice that your shoulders feel broader and your chest is open. You can breathe more fully. Your upper back is less rounded so that your neck flows easily upward into your skull. Your head is over your shoulders instead of forward in front of your neck. With your shoulders falling back and down, you can now access the muscles that connect your arms to your back.

Stand in front of a mirror. While drawing your upper arms backward into your shoulder sockets, pressing and lowering your shoulder blades down, note that the top of your arm moves just a little behind your chest. This was the position of your arms when you were lying on the rolled-up towel. When you let go of your shoulder blades and allow your chest to sink, your upper arm bones release forward. To keep your arms belonging to your back, you will need to train muscles to engage your shoulder blades.

Practice broadening your chest, drawing your upper arm bones back into your shoulder sockets, and sliding your shoulder blades down the sides of your back and away from your head. Your upper arms move slightly behind your chest. There is no need to arch your back. Isolate and gently activate your shoulder blades without forcing your rib cage forward. With your arms belonging to your back, you can allow your shoulders to hang like a clothes hanger, in alignment with your hips.

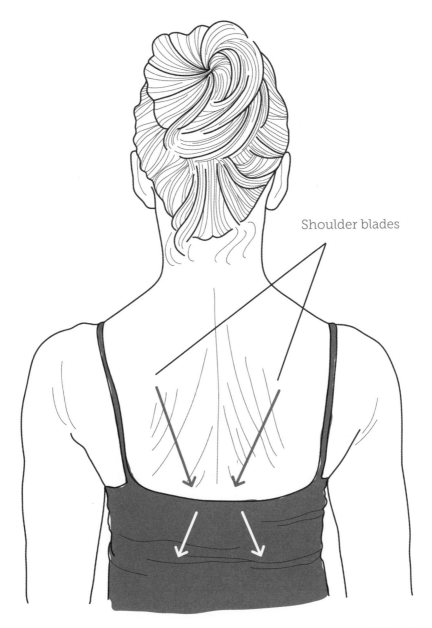

Shoulder blades

3. Abdominal Muscles Connect the Upper Body to the Lower Body

For optimal alignment and balance, your body needs a sense of unified wholeness. Unrelated pieces are hard to control. For instance, what connects the upper half of your body to the lower half? Is it only your back? The answer is: no.

Too much use of your back—contracting your lower back muscles for stability and to stand up straight—inactivates your abdominal muscles in the front of your body. For the purposes of this book, where, as we have discussed, your arms belong to your back, think of your abdomen as connecting your upper body to your lower body. You may need help finding that connection. Be patient with yourself.

Lie on your back on the floor, with your knees bent and soles of your feet on the floor. Feel your spine as long and relaxed, your head and tailbone as heavy at either end. Lower your shoulders away from your ears and allow them to fall toward the floor, behind your chest. Spread your hands on your lower abdomen, palms flat, the fingertips of each hand facing each other. Close your eyes and observe your breathing.

When you breathe in, your abdomen expands and rises; when you breathe out, your abdomen naturally falls and narrows. Feel the movement. On your inhale, the fingertips of your right hand move apart from those of your left hand. As you exhale, when your belly has relaxed all the way down, your fingertips will touch or intermingle.

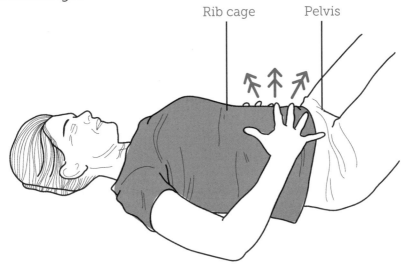

Rib cage   Pelvis

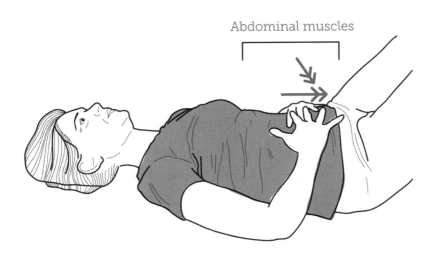

Abdominal muscles

At the end of the exhalation, let your abdominal muscles sink and firm further toward the floor. Now, squeeze out even more air. Bring your belly to your back and your sides toward the center. You're lightly using your abdominal muscles. Don't let your belly push out and don't tighten your chest. You won't need your neck, shoulders, back, or buttocks, either—those are the wrong muscles for the job. Relax your neck, shoulders, back, and buttocks part by part and keep them soft so that you isolate your abdominals.

With your hands on your abdomen, you can feel your bottom ribs travel toward your lower belly as your abdominal muscles firm and flatten. Your navel sinks back to the floor, too. Below your navel, the muscles harden as your belly sinks more. It's not a lot of work. Actually, the hardest part is relaxing everything else! By activating your abdominal muscles, the falling movement of your rib cage in the front, toward your pelvis and the lower body, is connecting your upper body to your lower body.

Now, stand up and do the same abdominal exercise with your hands on your lower belly, fingertips of your right hand toward those of the left hand. Inhale to feel relaxed expansion of your abdomen. Exhale to gently press the full front of your abdomen back toward your spine. The bottom of your rib cage will move a little

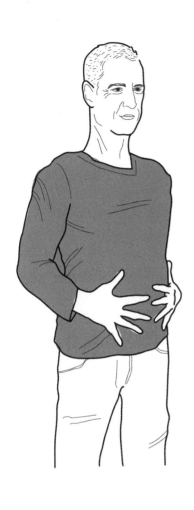
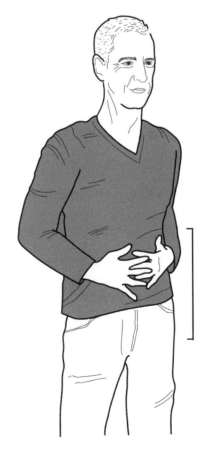

Connect upper body and lower body

toward your legs and your pelvis will link to your upper body.

Note the subtle feeling of connecting your pelvis to your upper body. Your center of gravity is inside your lower pelvis, so you can think of that center as the connection. The supportive feeling of that connection is your abdominal muscles unifying your torso, with its relaxed spine and open chest, on top of your legs.

To finish up, walk around a bit, relaxed and breathing, engaging and sinking your abdomen toward the back of your body, keeping everything else easy. Sense your upper body calmly connected to your center of gravity, low in the pelvis, so that your torso has a front-body feeling of unity over your legs.

You can stand tall and broad, without hunching, and move freely, connected in the front by your abdominal muscles.

4. The Secret of Youth Is a Long Front Body

A lifetime of sitting has deadened the nerves and muscles of your derriere. Even when you stand up, your buttocks muscles may still be turned off. Those muscles need to be activated so you can walk with your torso on top of your legs.

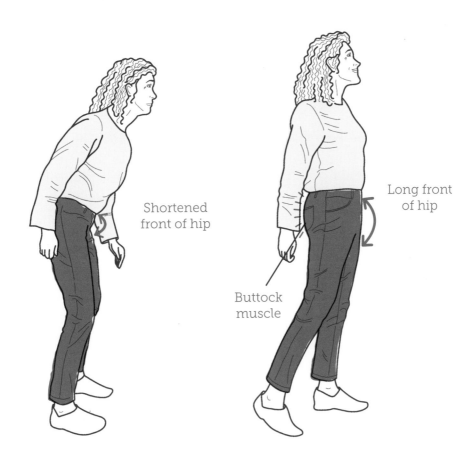

Shortened front of hip

Long front of hip

Buttock muscle

Try this experiment: Hinge forward from where your torso meets your legs to make a bent angle at the hips. From this position, try to contract your buttocks. Now, pull your body up on top of your legs so as to lengthen the front of your hips. Again, contract your buttocks. Which position makes it easier to feel your buttocks muscles engage? These muscles need to be accessible so they can do their work at the hip. The secret of youth is a long front body. Let's find length in front of your hips.

Lie on your back on the floor with your lower legs up on the seat of a chair, so that your hips and knees are bent at 90-degree angles.

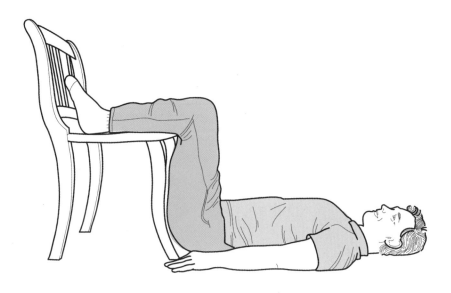

Slide the back of your head away from your hips and feel the length of your spine with weight at the very end of your tailbone. Relax your whole back. Breathe here for several minutes while you settle into the pull of gravity. The back of your neck or waist may not touch the floor; let those areas be light. This is your neutral spine. If your chin is up and the back of your neck feels constricted, place a slim book beneath your head.

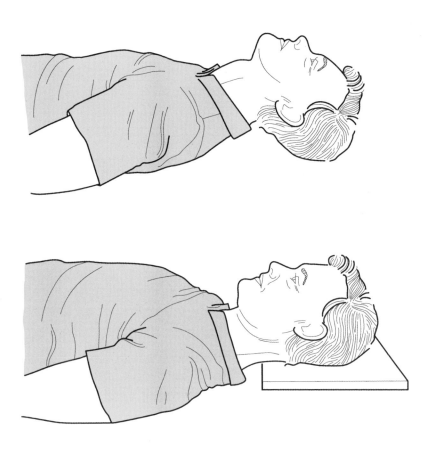

Now, move the chair slightly to the right so that you continue to rest your right leg at a 90-degree angle on the chair. Lower your left foot onto the floor and slowly extend your leg to its full length along the floor. Do you feel a stretch in front of the left hip? You will also notice the back of your left leg gradually falling closer to the floor. This could take several minutes. Continue to relax your back into a neutral position.

After you can feel the back of your left thigh and knee against the floor, change sides. Move the chair to the left and place your left leg back up on the chair seat at a 90-degree angle. Lower your right foot onto the floor so your right leg can slowly extend to its full length. Don't use force to make your right hip extend. Simply allow the weight of your leg to create the stretch in front of your right lower abdomen, hip, and upper thigh.

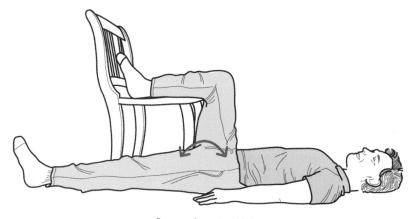

Long front of hip

After experiencing a satisfying stretch for the front of both hips, stand up and notice that your torso feels higher on top of your legs. Your front body is longer. Now that your hips are extended, you can better use your buttocks muscles. Contract your right and left buttocks just to prove they can be activated.

Use your new long front body to practice walking. With each step forward, imagine that you are pushing the ground behind you, using the strength of your buttocks. You will alternate right- and left-hip buttock contractions as you alternate legs. Don't forget the abdominal connection between your upper and lower body!

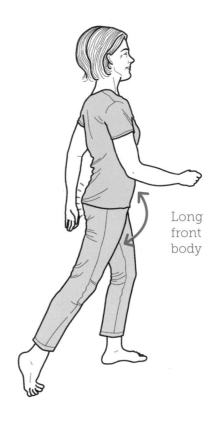

Long front body

5. The Feet Articulate

If your feet were as stiff as blocks of wood, they would not serve as a good base for balancing or an easy walking stride. Without flexible feet, you would have to depend more on your thighs and the front of your hips to walk.

Articulation, or joint mobility, of your foot gives you the power to push off from the front of your foot, or forefoot, and your big toe. This push propels your body forward so that walking is falling forward from one foot to the next.

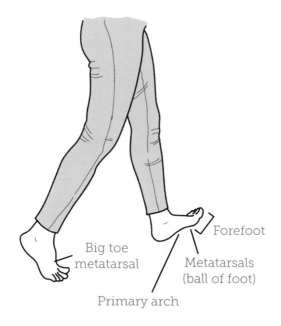

Forefoot

Big toe
metatarsal

Metatarsals
(ball of foot)

Primary arch

Heel-ball-toe mobility

Relaxed micro-movements of the foot are an important part of standing and balancing. As in walking, if your feet lack mobility, other parts of your body may be working too hard to compensate for a too rigid base. It will be much harder to balance.

Find a tennis ball, or even better, a solid rubber ball of about that size. Place it on the floor and stand where you can touch sturdy furniture or a wall for support. Position your right foot on top of the ball, with the ball under your forefoot. The joints at the base of your toes and part of your forefoot, the metatarsal bones, will take a dome shape from the ball underneath. Gradually transfer your body weight over the ball, allowing the metatarsals to mold to the shape of the ball. It may not feel entirely pleasant at first, so take it easy and go slowly. For one minute, maintain a bearable amount of

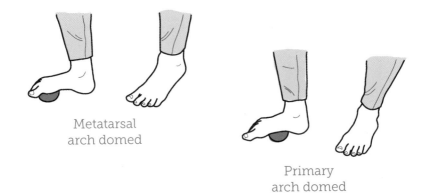

Metatarsal
arch domed

Primary
arch domed

your body weight over your forefoot while it is cupped and pressing the ball.

Now, roll the ball directly under the center of your foot and its primary arch. Gradually put weight onto the ball, or as much weight as you can tolerate. For one minute, maintain a bearable amount of your body weight over your arch while it is mashing the ball.

After you have released the stiffness from the bottom of your right foot, take your foot off the ball and stand on the floor. Your toes may feel straighter and longer. Your foot will feel wide, long, and grounded, providing a better base. Give your left foot the same treatment.

After you have pressed and massaged the bottom, or plantar surfaces, of your feet in this way, you can stand with a solid connection to your newly articulate feet. Walk around the room without shoes. With increased flexibility, your feet will feel more active with each step. Articulate feet have more than flexibility; they have enhanced power.

Become more sensitive to the actions of your feet. Stand with equal weight on both feet and shift your weight forward and backward from toes to heels. Shift from side to side as well. How does it feel when your weight shifts to the inside of the foot? Or to have most of your weight on the outside of the foot? Try moving your weight around in a circle while bringing your center of gravity over your ankles.

Distribute your weight over a tripod composed of your big toe, little toe, and heel. Although your feet are your base, notice the connections and adjustments happening in your whole body. This awareness will serve you well as we approach the 10 Weeks of Daily Activities to improve your balance.

10 Weeks of
Daily Activities

The information given in the opening sections will help you understand and approach the activities in the upcoming ten-week plan. As you work through the moves, you can always refer back for guidance, so let's start!

Follow the progression so that each week and its activities will build the skills you need for the following week. You won't need special clothes because these activities can be done alongside your daily routines. As you wait for the microwave, there is "Kitchen Counter Flat Back." Practice the "Shower Chest Stretch" when you wash your hair. Your morning cup of coffee or tea will serve as the cue for "Cup of Coffee Seated Shoulder Blade Retraction." Watch for Your Walking Stride prompts to help improve your gait. Some weeks have downtime activities that are productive ways to use TV-watching or help you unwind at the end of the day.

Don't be discouraged if, with your first attempt, you don't achieve the position shown in an illustration. In time you will acquire the flexibility or strength to perform the maneuver and benefit from the process of getting there. If the activities in a given week seem especially pertinent to your own physical issues, don't hesitate to repeat that week—or select and repeat the activities that seem most helpful.

Most of all, you needn't feel frustrated with what you may perceive as a failure to balance in the activity prescribed. With a secure fixture well within your reach, patiently steady yourself with the lightest motion you can to regain balance, then ease back into the balance challenge again. Even if you lose your equilibrium, you succeed in turning on your balance system and achieve the goal of practicing balancing. In fact, while practicing, teetering out of the balance is a great rehearsal for a surprise loss of balance in the course of daily life. You are better able to cope because your body knows what to do from experience. When you stand in an unstable position, sensory nerve endings that give information about your body's position and movement are getting the stimulation and practice they need to stay functional. In a strange way, experiencing losing your balance is the goal.

With that aim, keep in mind that every time you attempt an activity and "fail" to maintain your balance, you have in fact succeeded. Relax and try the activity again the next day.

Anxiety and tension are the enemies. Take it easy. If your feet tighten during a move, massage and release tension in your foot with the tennis ball as suggested in "The Feet Articulate" (page 30). If all seems lost when you close your eyes in a balance, take care to keep one finger lightly touching a sturdy base. Give yourself time to adapt to the lack of visual orientation.

The goal throughout the ten weeks is to accumulate your own repertory of training cues—the movement awareness activities and balances that stay with you for the future. After completing the ten-week plan, circle back to the moves from one of the early weeks and see how much easier they feel!

Week 1

What better place to start balance practice than
by lying in bed. I promised you this would be
easy! Important to good balance is stretching and
lengthening key parts of the body. This can be done
anywhere. Let's begin.

1. The Big X in Bed

In the morning when you wake up, squirm around using your whole body—limbs, spine, hips, rib cage, and neck. Take in deep breaths through your nose and out through your mouth.

Lie on your back in the middle of your bed with your right hand reaching diagonally toward the right upper corner of the bed and your left hand reaching toward the left upper corner. Spread your legs downward and out diagonally toward the right and left lower corners, so your body makes the shape of an X.

Lead with your right hand, palm down, to slide across your body until it makes contact with your left palm. The rest of your body will turn sequentially toward the left.

Keep your right leg in place, reaching toward the lower right corner of the bed. If you need to, hook your right foot around the edge of the mattress as you twist. Relax for a minute when you are settled all the way onto your left side, and feel the front of your right hip and abdomen stretching.

To do the same thing on the other side, make a big X and lead with your left hand across your body to your right palm. Now, leaving your left leg in place, stretch the front of the left side of your body.

Don't forget to breathe through the minute of stretching on each side. The secret of youth is a long front body. Be aware of that length all week.

Afterward, hug your knees to round your back.

If someone else shares your bed, then you can do "The Big X" on a floor rug.

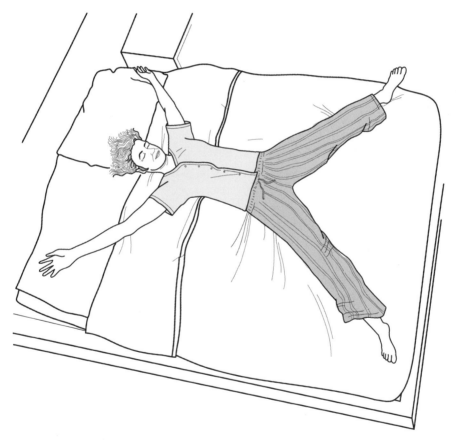

The Big X in Bed, starting position

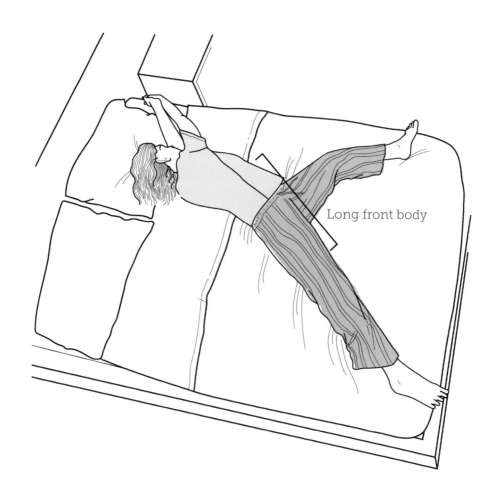

Long front body

The Big X in Bed, ending position

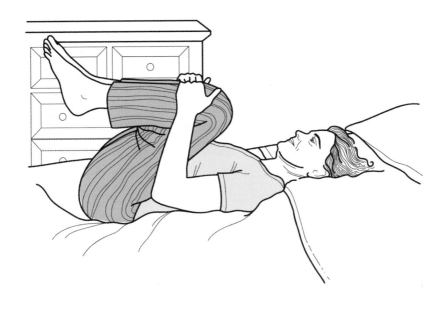

The Big X in Bed, back release

2. Kitchen Counter Flat Back

Whenever you wait for the water to boil, the toaster to toast, or the microwave to heat, take a moment to stretch the back of your body. Stand with the front of your body touching the kitchen counter. Put your hands on the kitchen counter and step away slowly as you lean forward until your back is flat and at a 90-degree angle to your legs (or as close as you can comfortably come to a right angle).

You will be in the shape of an L, legs perpendicular to the floor. Spread your fingers and reach your arms away from your hips while the tail end of your spine reaches in the opposite direction, away from your fingertips. Feel your back getting longer and imagine your breath flowing in between each bone of your spinal column.

If you can't get your back flat, or feel uncomfortable, then bend your knees. If your back feels long and flat, then try straightening your legs. You are stretching to feel the length of your entire back body, including the back of your legs.

To come out of the stretch without putting your back at risk for strain, keep your hands on the countertop and

walk all the way in toward the counter before you roll
your spine up to vertical position.

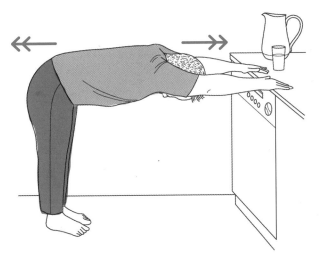

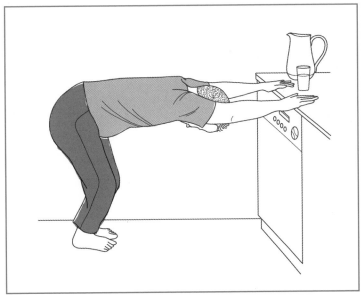

Try bending your knees

3. Toilet Lid Stance

When you're in the bathroom, close the lid of the toilet and take a moment to put your right leg up on the seat with your knee bent and your foot flat on the lid. Stand tall on your left leg and allow the right leg to make a 90-degree angle from your thigh to your torso.

Keep your hips level with each other and squarely facing the foot on the lid of the john. You are pretty much standing on one leg, so make sure you are situated so you can touch a wall or bathroom counter if you need to steady yourself.

Feel your long front body at the front of the left hip, just as it feels in "The Big X" (page 40). Let your right hip bend and relax downward. Don't tense the standing foot. Lengthen your toes going forward and your heel going backward in the opposite direction.

Sense your weight over a tripod of your big toe, little toe, and heel. Be calm and breathe for one minute. Your spine hangs free from your head like the string on a floating helium balloon.

Next time you're in the bathroom, put your left leg up in the same manner so you can feel the length of your right front body and allow the left hip to fall and bend easily.

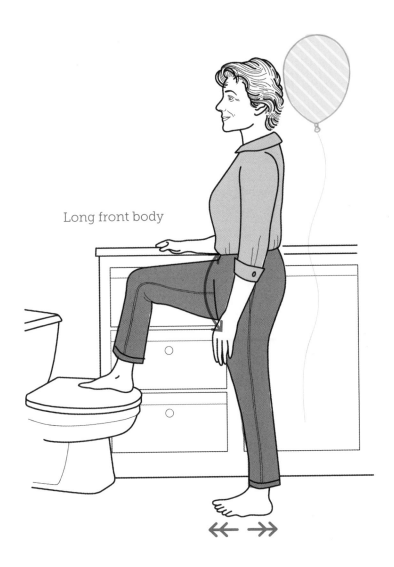

Long front body

Helium Balloon

Since gait disorders are a predictor of falling, it's well worth examining how you walk—and exploring how you can unify your body mechanics to walk more powerfully. Watch for Your Walking Stride tips during the ten-week plan.

This first week, when you are walking, use the image of a helium balloon as the back of your head, behind your ears—not under your chin—so that the back of your neck lengthens and your head floats back and up instead of sinking forward. Imagine that your cheekbones are sliding slightly backward, in the direction of behind your shoulders. A lifestyle of driving, gazing at a screen, and rounding your shoulders may have deflated your head balloon and compressed the back of your neck. This forward head position inhibits the spinal movement needed for a healthy striding gait. Walk and signal the adjustment of your head and neck relationship with the cue "helium balloon."

4. Shower Chest Stretch

While standing in the shower, face the showerhead and extend your right arm behind you along the shower wall to your right at three o'clock, palm flat on the wall. Feel a stretching sensation in front of your right chest. Let the warm water relax your shoulders downward.

Allow your neck to grow upward into your skull and the helium balloon at the back of your head to float upward. Connect your upper body to your lower body by gently sinking your front bottom ribs downward toward your abdomen and your abdomen into your pelvis.

Turn around and face the opposite direction or switch sides, so that your left arm extends behind you on the shower wall, palm flat, at nine o'clock. Now you are stretching your left chest muscles.

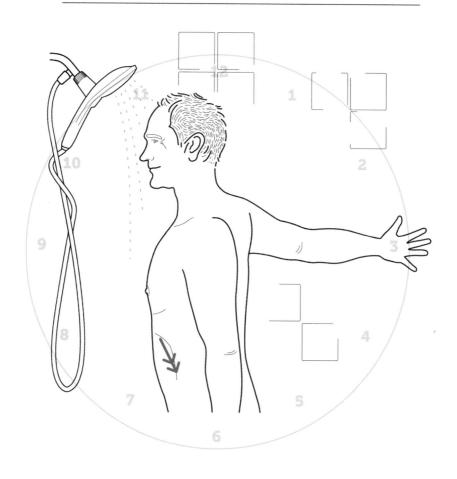

Shower Chest Stretch

Attention to Your Feet: After you've showered or bathed, sit down and dry in-between your toes with a towel. Stretch each toe away from the others for individual consideration. Think of your feet as capable of the same span and dexterity as your hand. This open base of support will be your foundation for next week's balancing activities.

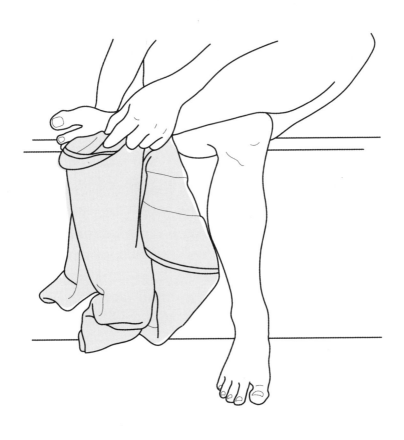

Habit Alert

Committing to this ten-week plan is a fresh start for you. It's time to do things differently. This week, when you put on your shirt or jacket, instead of putting the same arm in the sleeve first as you usually do, stop yourself, and put the other arm in first. Give the other side of your body a chance to make the first move and get the same flexibility and joint action the leading arm has developed over time. It's good for both brain and body.

Week 2

Last week you stretched and increased your body's range. During this second week, you will activate muscles to support your new, extended body—and posture.

1. Cup of Coffee Shoulder Blade Retraction

Each morning this week, while sitting at the table with your coffee, tea, or breakfast, use muscles in your back to move your shoulder blades. Remember, your arms belong to your back—not to your neck and chest.

First, exaggerate rounding your shoulders forward and sinking your chest to feel compression at the back of your neck. To reverse this effect, broaden your chest and think of drawing your upper arms back into your shoulder sockets. Slide your shoulder blades down the sides of your back and away from your head. Now, relax your neck. Feel it release upward into your skull so that the back of your head floats.

Notice that as you engage and retract your shoulder blades into position, your upper arms move backward. As they join with your shoulder blades moving down your back, relax your rib cage.

Notice the same openness in your chest, in front of your right and left shoulders, that you felt in the "Shower Chest Stretch" from last week (page 49).

Do the shoulder blade retraction ten times.

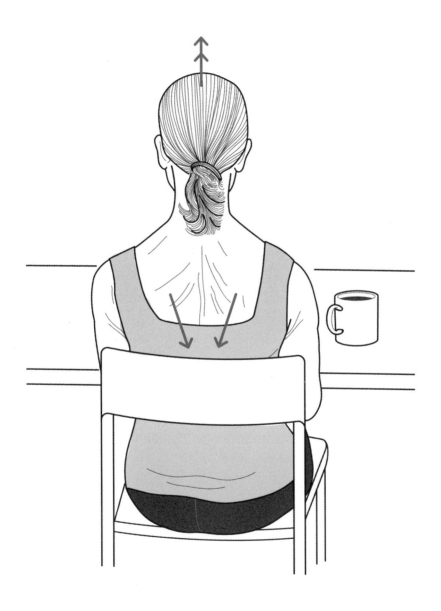

2. Brushing Teeth Balance No. 1— Finger Touching Base

Each time you brush your teeth, morning and night, steady yourself by placing your fourth (ring) finger of the non-toothbrush-holding-hand on the edge of the sink or bathroom counter. Move one foot slightly behind you and off the floor. Stand on one leg while keeping the fourth finger on the sink edge.

Even with the one finger on the sink you might lose your balance, so be ready to touch the foot down to rest your toe on the floor until you feel steadier; you can then take the foot back off the floor to continue balancing while you brush your teeth. Keep the fourth finger on the sink or counter edge at all times.

Don't worry if you lose your balance. If you need to, just keep resting the toe of the nonstanding foot on the floor. This balance may take some time and practice.

Alternate the standing leg for morning and night brushing.

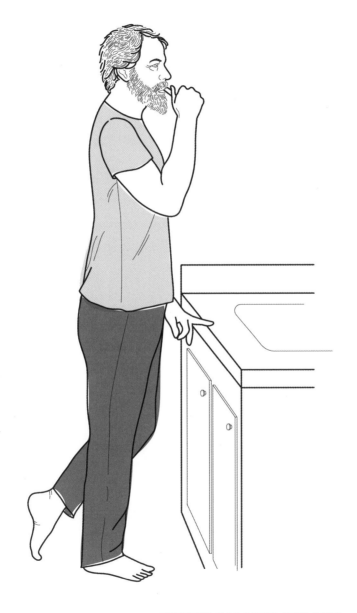

3. Sit-to-Stand Squat No. 1— Using Arms

We all stand up from sitting many times a day. This week, use careful form to activate your buttocks muscles and "squat up."

Scoot the chair back, if necessary, and slide to the front of the seat, placing both feet flat on the floor about hips–width apart. While remaining seated, contract your buttocks muscles and keep them contracted.

Now, lean forward, relaxing your head to fall forward slightly, and shift your center of gravity over your ankles as you take weight onto both feet. Watch that your kneecaps bend and point in the same direction as your toes—not to the insides of your feet. Use your arms, either on the arms of the chair or on your thighs, to help support your weight as you squat up. Don't try to lift yourself up using your back muscles. Use your already contracted buttocks and your thighs to do the work as you come to standing.

Use the same form in reverse each time you sit down.

Don't forget to use every opportunity of sitting down or standing up to practice the correct form for squat-down or squat-up.

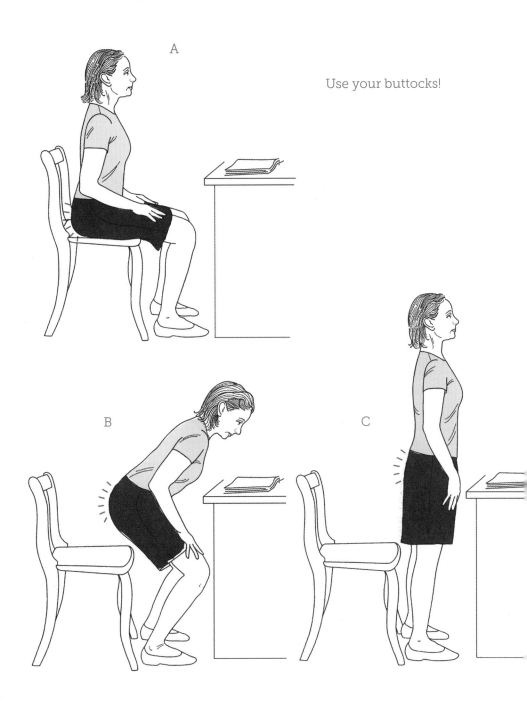

A

Use your buttocks!

B

C

A Rear that's in Gear: Use your buttocks muscles to stand up and sit down; not your back muscles. Can't feel your buttocks working when you sit down or stand up? Get the muscles activated before the squat up or squat down so they will know what to do.

Let's practice. When sitting, isolate and contract your buttocks. This action will lift your sitting position slightly higher onto the contracted muscle. Feel the shift. Keep the contraction and explosively propel yourself to standing so the buttocks don't have time to let go!

Now practice squatting down from standing to sitting. Contract the buttocks while standing. Don't change your posture, just feel your butt powerfully isolated. Commit to the contraction and don't let go until you are sitting on a chair, on top of your contracted buttocks. Finally, you can release them. Once you have the knack you won't have to try so hard. Your butt will automatically kick in to assist your strengthening thighs and eliminate undue stress on your knees.

4. Television Time— Mind-to-Foot Control

You've used muscle power to stabilize your shoulders. You powered your hips to squat up to standing. Now, let's work your feet.

While watching TV, take off your shoes and interlace your fingers with your toes to separate them. (Last week's shower activity of towel drying in-between your toes stretched your toes apart, so now they will accept your interlaced fingers more readily.)

After that preparation, prop one foot on the coffee table or couch and spread all five toes so no toe touches another. Fan the toes in this way ten times for each foot.

Alternate pointing your foot, extending your toes away from your face, then flexing your ankle, drawing the toes toward your face. Use this three-part heel-ball-toe sequence: (A) extend the ankle, (B) push through to the ball (metatarsal) of the foot with your toes still flexed toward your face, and (C) extend your toes. Return to the starting position in reverse order, flexing the toes *only* at first and then through the foot to the ankle. Do the three-part extension and flexion ten times for each foot.

Now wiggle one toe at a time, from the big toe to the little toe. At first you may not be able to get your mind to connect to your foot very well, but it will get better as you progress through the week. Relax the rest of your body while you focus on your foot. Don't try to move your toes with your knee, hip, or face!

Repeat the sequence with the other foot.

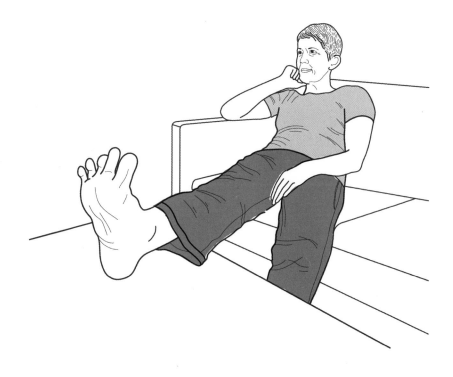

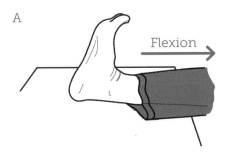

A

Flexion →

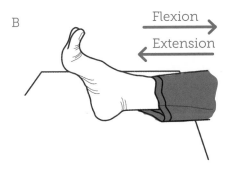

B

Flexion →
← Extension

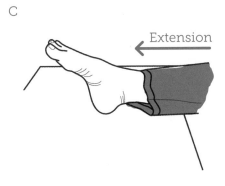

C

← Extension

Reverse the sequence: C, B, and back to A

Big Toe Push Off/ Falling Forward

Liberate your feet. Walk around the house barefoot as much as you can this week. Without the restriction of shoes, feel the twenty-six bones in each foot moving freely while your feet make contact with the floor.

As you swing your leg through to take a step forward, flex your ankle and turn your toes up toward your face. This action will keep your foot from dropping and potentially causing you to stumble. Although you should consider the arch of the foot as reaching forward, you will notice that your heel hits the ground first. Exaggerate the separate heel-ball-toe actions—the ones you used while watching TV—as you strike the heel and roll through your foot on the floor. Finally, push the floor behind you with your toes.

Walking about during your week, give yourself the cue "big toe push off" and prompt "falling forward" to mobilize your feet that send you forward from one foot to the other.

You now have two cues for Your Walking Stride: "helium balloon" and "big toe push off/falling forward."

Week 3

Last week you activated muscles in your shoulders, buttocks, and feet. Use this new feeling of power to ground your legs and stand stronger.

1. Brushing Teeth Balance No. 2— No Hands!

Building on Brushing Teeth Balance No. 1 from the previous week, stand on one leg with your fourth finger on the sink edge.

As you begin brushing your teeth, slowly take your finger off the sink. Touch your non-standing toe down to the floor to keep steady anytime you need to. You can keep your foot there as long as you want. But try not to use your hand or finger on the bathroom counter for balance.

Even if your foot wobbles, think of spreading the standing tripod—big toe, little toe, and heel—on the floor. Press downward with your weight through the big toe metatarsal. Remember how you engaged your buttocks muscles to stand from the chair last week in "Sit-to-Stand Squat" (page 58)? Now you can access your buttocks muscle to stabilize your hip over your standing leg.

Using opposing forces, reach down through your leg to the floor, as your spine and head float upward in the opposite direction.

Avoid tensing or gripping muscles. Instead, focus on reaching muscles into stabilizing length and strength.

Stand on the other leg when you brush your teeth at night.

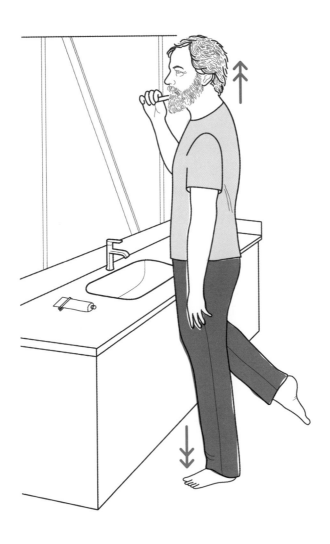

2. Rinsing Dishes Heel Raises

Whenever you find yourself at the kitchen sink, stand with your feet hips-width apart and parallel to each other. Rest your forearms on the sink while you work, so you feel steady.

Push downward through the big toe metatarsals of your forefeet as you gradually lift your heels off the floor. You don't need to lift them as high as you can. The first days of the week, lift your heels halfway to their full height capacity.

The raised heels are not dangling in space—they are level with each other and you are aware of their relation to the floor.

Work up to raising and lowering your heels twenty times. Afterward, stretch your lower leg muscles with "Cookbook Calf Stretch."

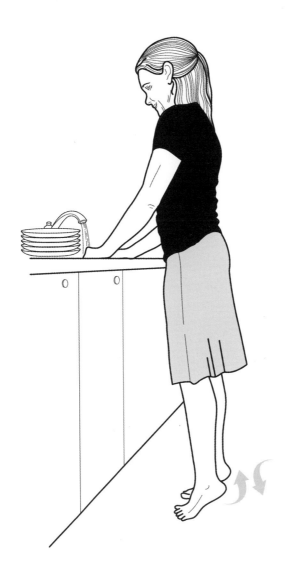

Cookbook Calf Stretch: After your work at the kitchen sink, place a sturdy, thick cookbook on the floor. Place both forefeet on the book with your heels hanging off so that, eventually, the heels rest on the floor. Breathe as you stand in the position for a while. Imagine your calf muscles are descending as they stretch.

Avoid bending at the hips. Stand with your long front body, raising your hips directly on top of your legs. Allow your front ribs to relax down into the front of your pelvis. Retract your shoulder blades so that your upper arms connect to your back, as in "Cup of Coffee Shoulder Blade Retraction" (page 54).

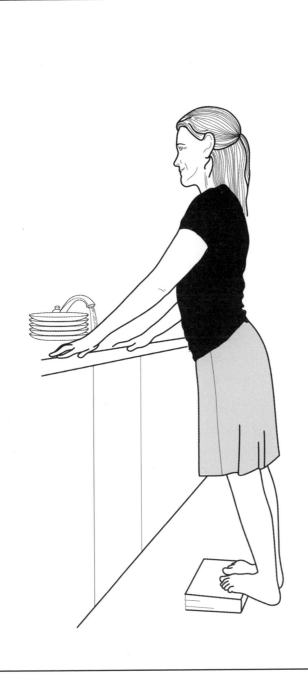

3. Phone Stance No. 1—Shin Bones Press In

Stand up each time you text or talk on the phone to practice engaging your legs for enhanced stability. With your feet hips-width apart and all ten toes relaxed straight ahead, imagine a balloon placed between your lower legs. Press the insides of your shins toward each other to squeeze the imaginary balloon. Your right shin moves to the left and your left shin moves to the right. With this action, you activate your legs and hips, connecting the big-toe metatarsals of your forefeet with the floor. At the same time, maintain weight on your little toes and your heels. Your hips and knee caps face straight ahead. Be mindful of your long front body, with your hips on top of your legs.

As you use your phone throughout the day, practice pressing your shin bones in on the imaginary balloon. Use the engagement of your legs as if to lift the balloon all the way up the insides of your legs. In this way, connect your lower body to your upper body. Hold your phone at eye level so that your head can float back and up, not forward and down.

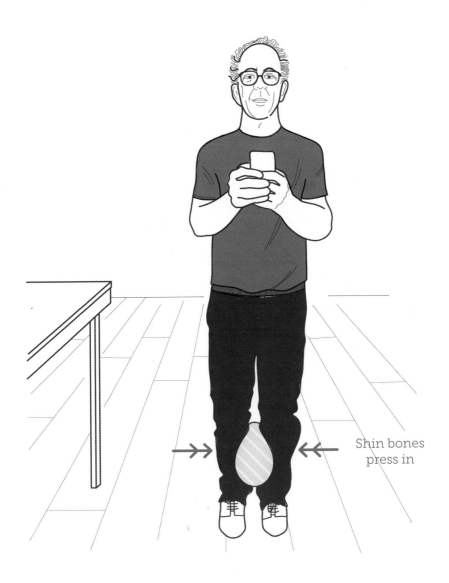

Shin bones
press in

Habit Alert

Your body mechanics are changing. Shake up old habits. If you routinely use a shoulder bag, carry it on the opposite shoulder this week. If you carry a briefcase or handheld tote, hold it in the opposite hand.

While carrying on either side, release your shoulders down, engage your shoulder blades in your back with symmetrical strength, and lighten the back of your head.

You will have to resist the urge to switch the bag to the habitual side. Try sustaining the nonhabitual side for longer periods of time as the week goes on. If you prefer, convert to using a backpack.

4. Over the Rainbow Against the Wall

Now that you are aware of your long front body, thanks to "The Big X" (page 40) and your long back body, thanks to "Kitchen Counter Flat Back" (page 44), it's time to stretch your side body as well.

Find an area of wall space in a room or hallway that you pass frequently. The wall could be where you wait for the elevator at work, or maybe there is sufficient space in a hallway in your home where you come and go regularly. Whenever you walk by that spot you can stretch the sides of your body with the following movement.

Stand with your back against the wall, heels several inches away from its base, knees relaxed. Feel the bottom tip end of your spine, your shoulders, the back of your elbows, the back of your hands, and even the back of your head against the wall. If you can't get the back of your head to touch the wall without shortening the back of your neck, then allow the helium balloon at the back of your head to float up without your head touching the wall. Don't strain. Think of sending the front of your torso toward the wall behind you.

Draw the shape of a rainbow on the wall, initiating the movement with your head leading to the right, so your spine follows as it curves to the right in an arc. Try to keep your shoulders and arms against the wall as you do this, imagining your head is falling toward a pot of gold.

Feel a comfortable stretch on the left side of your body. Now you're ready to arc left over the rainbow to the other pot of gold and stretch the right side of your body.

Continue bending right and left ten times, stretching upward over the top of the rainbow with the crown of your head and then dropping your head sideways at the pot of gold. Do this every time you pass the designated wall.

Go easy, and limit the range in the beginning of the week. Increase the range gradually by the end of the week.

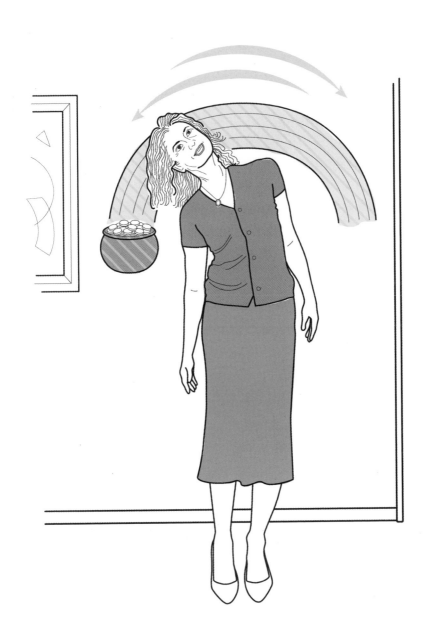

Towel Crumpling

Make a point to sit down and take a break at the end of each day this week. While doing something enjoyable like watching TV, having a conversation, or reading, you can relax and do some mindless footwork! Sit barefoot, feet placed on a smooth floor surface, hips-width apart. Set a dish towel on the floor to the outside of your left foot. Use your left toes and forefoot only, left heel resting on the floor, to crumple the towel along the floor toward your right foot. Once the entire towel is crimped and wrinkled to the right side of your left foot, you can pick it up with your hand, straighten it out, and return the towel to the starting position. Repeat several times, then do some towel crumpling on the other side with the right foot. Watch how it gets easier to do as the week goes by. Dexterous feet will be a boost to your balancing work in the weeks ahead.

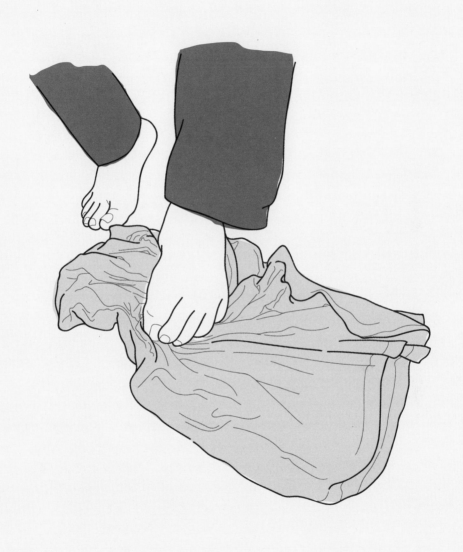

Week 4

After three weeks, you are well on the road to
better balance. Continue to practice balancing
and strengthen your lower body with heel raises
at the kitchen sink and by squatting to sit and
stand. Find more range of motion in your shoulder
joints by sweeping your arm on the wall like
the minute hand of a clock.

1. Brushing Teeth Balance No. 3—Arm Overhead

Are you feeling calmer about balancing on one leg? If so, hold your free arm overhead when you brush your teeth. Progress at your own pace. If you need more practice with Brushing Teeth Balance No. 2, continue doing it this week.

While extending one arm overhead, you will need to use your abdominal muscles to keep from leaning back. Don't let the reaching arm tilt your ribcage upward. Relax your bottom front ribs down into your pelvis. Deepen and firm your abdomen to connect upper body to lower body. At the same time, grow upward through your spine. Remember the opposing forces from last week. You grounded your standing leg on the floor while you let the back of your head rise like a helium balloon.

Reminder: Touch your toe to the floor to regain balance whenever necessary.

Alternate the standing leg for morning and night brushing. When you stand on your right leg, press your right shin to the left like you did while squeezing the imaginary balloon in "Phone Stance No. 1—Shin

Bones Press In" (page 72). When you stand on your left leg, press your left shin to the right. The resulting engagement will provide greater stability for standing on one leg.

Afterward, stretch the back of your thighs.

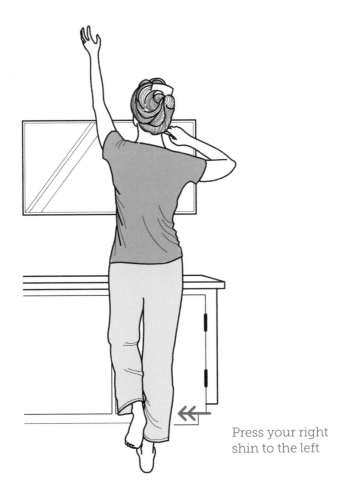

Press your right shin to the left

Back of Thigh Stretch: Stand upright facing the toilet with the vertical alignment of your cheekbones squarely over your two shoulders, and your shoulders over your hips. Prop the back of your right heel on top of the closed toilet lid with your ankle flexed, toes pointing up to the ceiling; both legs straightening.

Your spine is neutral, not hunched.

To keep your propped leg straight, firm the thigh muscles of the front of your right leg as if to draw your kneecap upward away from your knee and toward your hip. Keep the right hip down and pushed back behind you, not hitched upward, and feel a stretch behind the thigh of your right leg. Take ten slow breaths. Switch to standing on your right leg and propping the left leg on the toilet lid to stretch the back of your left thigh.

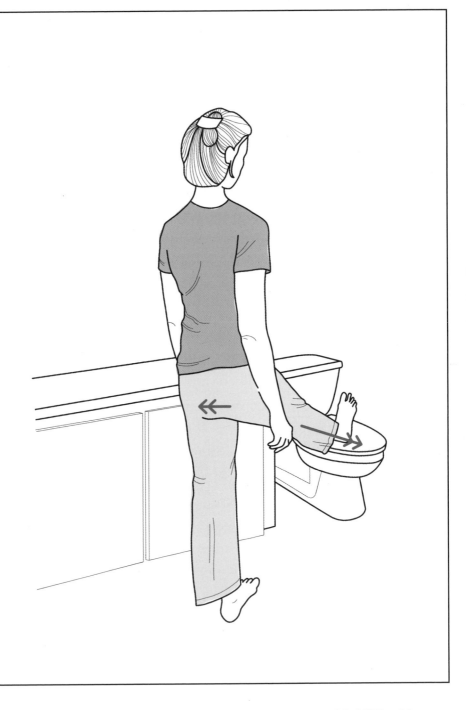

Shoulder Swagger

Marching is a good release after standing on one leg for too long. After you finish brushing your teeth and stretching your thigh, march in place to loosen up. When the right knee lifts, turn your shoulders to the right and touch your left hand to your right knee. When the left knee lifts, turn your shoulders to the left and touch your right hand to your left knee. In other words, twist toward the leading leg. Your arm should swing forward easily along with the opposite leg.

When you walk in the coming days and weeks, notice the subtle tendency of your shoulders to rotate in this way. Exaggerate the twist to feel the rotation more strongly. Let your arms swing. This natural "cross-crawl" encourages a pivoting in the spine and strengthens your nervous system and brain development, too! If you find that you are holding your shoulders and arms still and unconsciously inhibiting rotation of your spine, think: four-legged animal. You aren't walking with just your legs and feet; it's a total body movement that helps link your upper body with your lower body.

Cue cross-crawl shoulder rotation with the words "shoulder swagger." Now you have accumulated three cues for Your Walking Stride: "helium balloon,"

"shoulder swagger," and "big toe push off/falling forward."
Practice putting them all together as you walk.

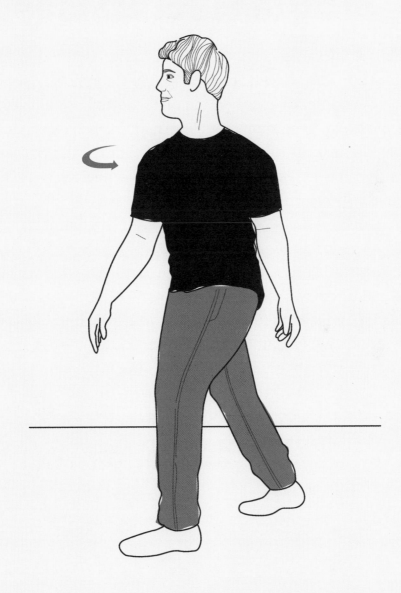

2. Rinsing Dishes Single Heel Raises

This is the same as last week's heel raises, but now you stand on just one leg at a time to repeat ten heel raises on the right foot and then ten on the left foot. You may not be able to do many repetitions at first because this requires significant strength from the single leg. Start with just three or four very small single heel raises and gradually work up to ten.

Lightly rest your forearms on the sink to maintain balance during the exercise. Relax your shoulders downward and maintain the good form you used while standing on two legs last week.

Explore feeling four corners of your standing foot on the floor: big toe, little toe, inner heel, outer heel. Your most important connection to the floor is the big-toe metatarsal of your forefoot. Press down through that connection to go up into the heel raise. It's opposing forces at work again.

If your calves feel tight, stand in "Cookbook Calf Stretch" (page 70).

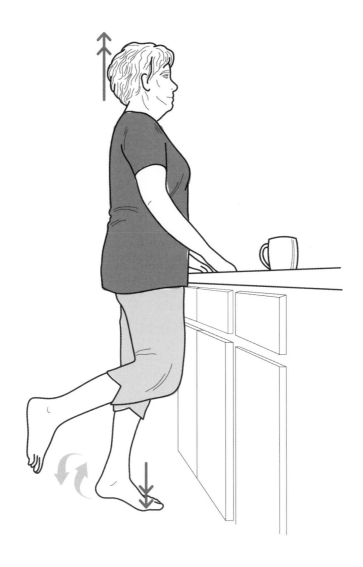

3. Sit-to-Stand Squat No. 2— Arms Crossed

Since you are now routinely squatting up from sitting to standing, and squatting down from standing to sitting, you are ready to intensify strengthening your lower body.

As in Week 2, each time you sit down or get up from a chair, prepare to squat up or squat down by placing your hips and feet appropriately.

This week, cross your arms over your chest so that when you rise, you do not use your hands on your thighs or on the arms of the chair.

In the squat, your weight will be supported by the lower body exclusively. If your legs and hips don't feel strong enough, keep just one arm crossed over your chest and try using one arm on your thigh to assist for a few days. If you need this support, alternate the arm you use to sit down or stand up.

Secure your heels on the floor. Contract your buttocks muscles while you are sitting *before* you stand up. Relax the front of your ankles and the back of your knees as you bend and fold into your ankle, knee, and hip joints. Transfer all your weight onto your legs. Continue contracting your buttocks to bring your hips over your legs.

Find a connection from your lower front rib cage through your abdomen into your pelvis so that your torso moves as one unit.

If you catch yourself improperly hefting yourself up with your back in the old way, sit back down and squat up with good form. The same is true for sitting down. If you plop down to take a seat with the back of your neck compressed or your ankles unbending, squat up, and squat back down correctly.

Without any help from your arms, performing these squats as part of your daily sitting and standing transitions, will strengthen your lower body and provide function for years to come.

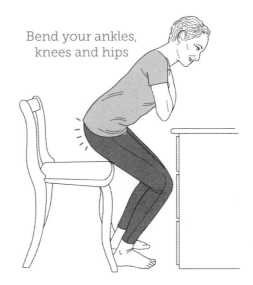

Bend your ankles, knees and hips

4. Minute Hand Sweeps the Clock at Wall

The same wall where you stopped to perform "Over the Rainbow Against the Wall" (page 75) is now your signal to do "Minute Hand Sweeps the Clock at Wall."

Stand with the wall at your left shoulder. Experiment to see how far from the wall you need to stand to successfully circle the long left arm with your fingertips grazing the wall, while you draw a circle.

Sweep your arm clockwise so that, like a minute hand, your fingers glide by each hour on the face of the clock eight times. You may be far away from the wall at first, drawing the circumference of a small clock. The closer you get to the wall, the bigger the clock will become and the greater the range of motion at the shoulder joint.

Relax the base of your neck and shoulder downward. Isolate your arm in its shoulder socket. Don't turn your body toward the wall as your arm circles. Keep your shoulders and hips squarely facing forward and perpendicular to the wall.

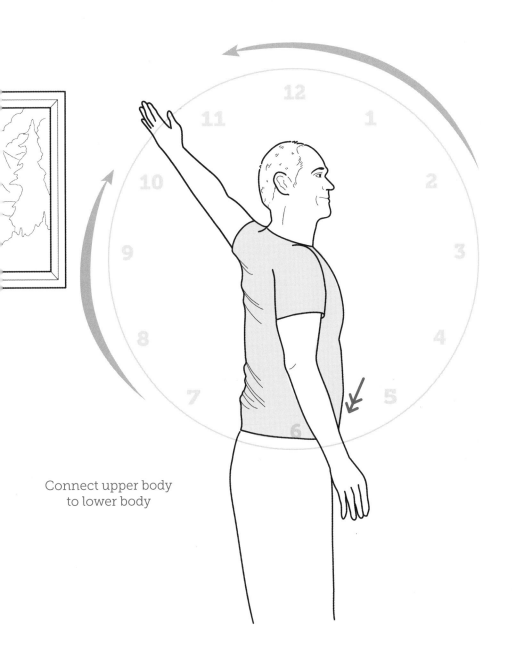

Connect upper body
to lower body

Reverse the circle so your right arm sweeps in a counterclockwise direction eight times. Turn around, face the other way, and circle your right arm both clockwise and counterclockwise eight times each direction.

You may have some difficulty when your right arm sweeps past two o'clock, and on the other side, when your left arm sweeps past ten o'clock. Slow down, breathe, and keep dropping your arm downward into its shoulder socket while your hand leads. Feel your shoulder blade moving fluidly in your back.

Passive Spiral Stretch

Here's your reward for the week. At the end of the day, let go of tense muscles. Healthy muscles relax and soften just as well as they contract and firm.

Lie on the floor and hug your knees to your chest to round your back. Keep your knees over your torso while you lower your arms out to the side and rest them wide on the floor at chest level. Secure the back of your left shoulder to the floor, and move both knees to the right. See whether your knees can reach the floor. If the twist is too great, put a cushion under or between your knees to lessen the range of the spiral.

Relax the weight of your legs onto the cushion or floor. Release your left shoulder toward the floor.

Slowly turn your head to the left.

Surrender your body into gravity. Inhale to expand into the stretch sensations of your entire left side. Use at least eight breaths to fall deeper into the pose with each exhalation.

Use your abdominal muscles, sinking and firming toward your spine, to anchor yourself as you move your bent legs toward your chest and over to the left for the opposite twist, keeping both arms on the ground.

Feel the stretch in front of your right shoulder and along your entire right side and, again, breathe yourself deeper into the passive stretch with every complete exhalation.

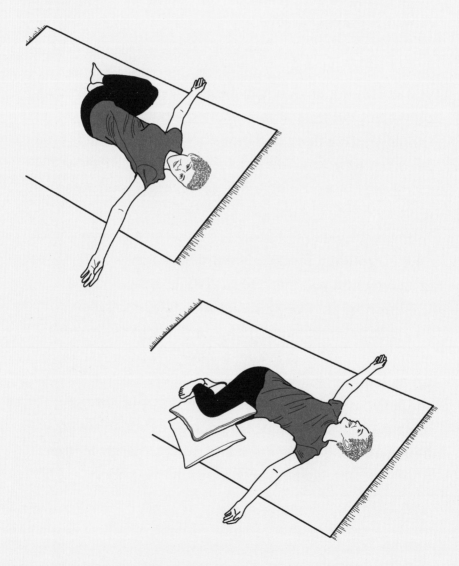

Week 5

It's the halfway week! Balance, step up, twist, and walk backward through your week.

1. Brushing Teeth Balance No. 4— One Eye Closed

If you are still working on "Brushing Teeth Balance No. 1" (page 56), that's fine. See whether you feel comfortable moving on to No. 2 (page 66). If you were doing No. 2 last week, try No. 3 (page 82). Progress at your own pace.

No. 4 is the same position as No. 2. Stand on one leg without touching the sink for support while you brush your teeth. As an added challenge, close one eye. Close the right eye in the morning when you stand on the left leg and close the left eye at night when you stand on the right leg.

Afterward, stretch the front of your thighs. Let go of tension in your body that you don't need and find the muscular engagement for stabilization that you *do* need.

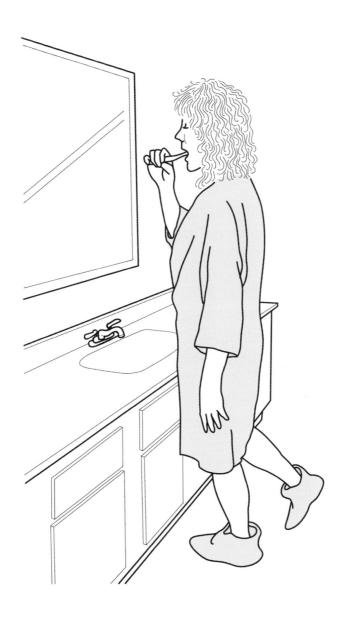

Front of Thigh Stretch: Face away from the toilet and prop the top of your left foot on the closed lid behind you, with your hand touching a sturdy stabilizer. Your left knee will be facing the floor. Stand upright on your right leg and you will feel a stretch in front of the left thigh that has the foot on the toilet seat.

Don't tense the stretching thigh. Imagine expanding the front of the stretching thigh with your inhalation and relaxing it with your exhalation. Make sure your pelvis is on top of your legs for a long front body. Keep both thighs and knees even with each other. Reverse to stretch the other side.

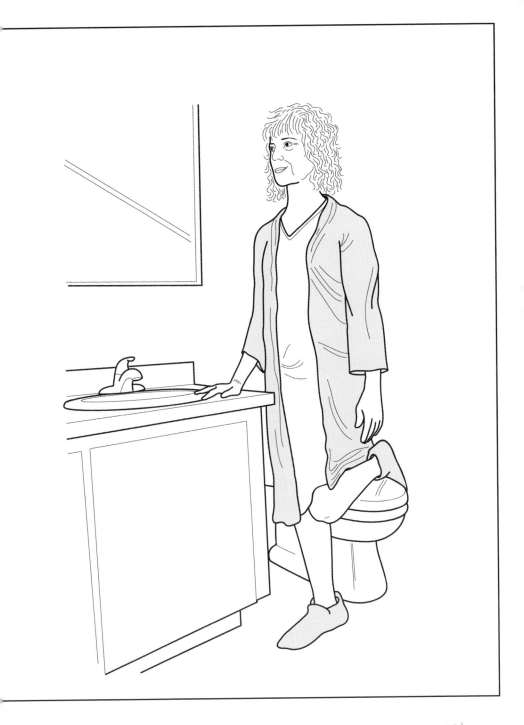

2. Step Up to Get Dressed No. 1— Touching Dresser

Place a low household step stool in front of your dresser. Each morning when you get dressed, practice stepping up on the step stool. Getting clothing out of a dresser drawer is your cue to do "Step Up to Get Dressed."

Face the dresser and put both hands lightly on it to steady yourself. Start with your right foot on the step in front of you, your weight on your left foot, which is on the floor behind the step.

Bend at your hips, knees, and ankles. Transfer your weight from your back left foot to the right foot on the step. Focus on the power of your right buttock muscle contracting so as to propel you forward and up onto the step. Pause as you stand on your right leg at the top of the step.

Then bend the ankle, knee, and hip of your right leg to lower yourself in preparation to descend backward and back onto your left leg. As you transfer weight through an articulate left foot, bend your left ankle, knee, and hip to cushion the landing.

Perform the step up and step down ten times while keeping your right foot on the step throughout. Reverse your starting position and keep your left foot on the step throughout.

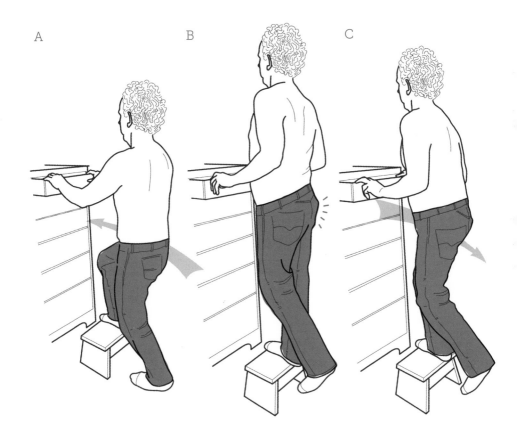

3. Mealtime Seated Twist in Chair

When you sit down at the table *before* a meal, twist your torso to strengthen and stretch postural muscles.

Sit sideways in a sturdy chair so that your feet and knees face a 90-degree angle away from the way you are supposed to sit. Feel your spine growing upward as you "perch" on top of your sitting bones. Allow the helium balloon at the back of your head to float up.

Twist toward the seat back and place one hand on each side of the seat back frame at about the level of your lower ribs.

Take a breath in. As you breathe out, turn your pelvis around in the direction of the twist without coming off your sitting bones. During the next exhalation, effortlessly revolve your rib cage around the axis of your spine. During the next exhalation, let your chest continue the spiral. Your range of motion will be small, but you can imagine a gentle whirlpool around your spine. Lastly, exhale to turn your shoulders. Don't lift your shoulders; let them relax. No need to twist your head and neck further.

Breathe into your back and keep growing upward out the crown of your head as you direct the tail end of your spine downward. Relax your abdomen. Don't force your way to a fixed end-point of the twist. Leave room for the feeling of endless rotation.

To repeat the twist in the other direction, sit with your feet and knees facing the opposite way.

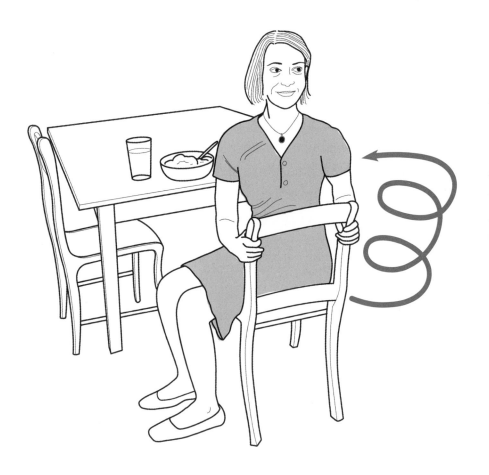

4. Walking Backward

Find a clear pathway in a room or hallway that will cue you to practice walking backward. Each time you go through the designated area, turn around and walk backward with a relaxed gait.

The first time, look behind you so you know how far to go. Count the steps so that in the future, without looking, you will know when to stop.

Be conscious of the transfer of weight in the less familiar stepping-backward walk and feel the reverse action of toe, ball, and heel stepping behind yourself. If you lose your balance, bend your ankles, knees, and hips to drop your weight lower into the ground.

The more you walk backward when you go through the designated area, the more confident, coordinated, and balanced you will become.

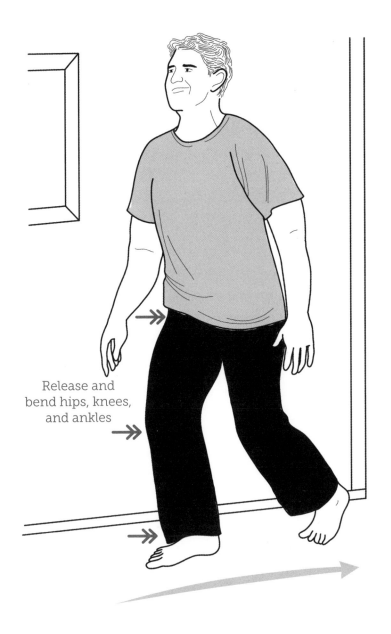

Release and
bend hips, knees,
and ankles

Bedtime Supported Bridge

As in previous weeks, use the end of the day to relax, breathe, and calm your body. At night, when you get into bed, lengthen your front body before you go to sleep.

Lying on your back with your knees bent and your feet flat on the bed, contract your buttocks to lift your pelvis high enough to put a pillow or two underneath your hips.

Once your hips are supported, slide your legs down and extend your arms overhead and comfortably out to the side. Relax for ten deep breaths.

Your body will arch like a bridge, with your arms and head at one end of the arc and your feet at the other end. Your pelvis is the apex. Feel the stretch sensation in the front of your upper thighs, hips, and lower abdomen.

If your lower back tightens, lengthen your pelvis further away from your back rib cage so that your lower back will be longer and relaxed.

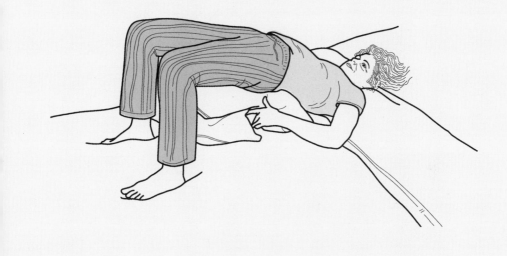

Stretching

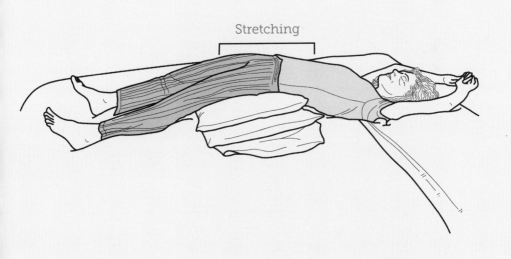

Week 6

Do you feel as if you've grown an inch in five weeks? You're more limber so that your body can release and grow and, at the same time, more compact so that your body can connect and ground in your balances.

1. Brushing Teeth No. 5—Teeter-totter

Keep doing whichever "Brushing Teeth" exercise you need to master next. If you feel good about No. 4 (page 98), then progress to No. 5.

While standing on one leg without touching the sink edge, pitch gently forward from your hips (at about a 45-degree angle) and allow the leg that is off the floor to move backward, as if your standing leg is the center of a teeter-totter. Your upper body, even though your torso is tilted from the hips, lifts through your chest to keep the spine long. Your back leg follows the same line of your spine like the plank of a seesaw, as you balance on one leg and brush your teeth.

When you need to spit into the sink, just teeter further forward, maintaining the diagonal line from your head to your back knee. When you are finished, use your buttock muscle to extend yourself back upright.

Change legs for night brushing.

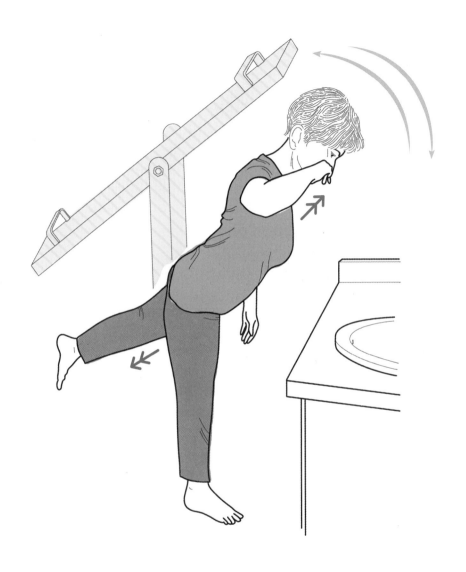

2. Putting on Socks No. 1—Wall Touch

Instead of sitting down to put on your socks, stand next to and barely touch your right shoulder to a wall, ready to put a sock on your left foot. The light touch of your shoulder or hip against the wall will provide support for standing on your right foot while you put your left foot into the sock and pull it on.

Try not to hunch your back. Keep in mind the growing length in the back of your neck, the shoulder-blade retraction that connects your arms into your back, and the abdominal muscles that connect the bottom of your ribs to your pelvis low in the front of your body.

Bend at your standing right ankle, knee, and hip to lower yourself closer to reach your left foot and put the sock on it. Direct your left hip downward as it bends to lift your left leg closer to your hands holding the sock. Keep your hips as level as possible.

Move slowly and be aware of the body mechanics involved as if you have never put on socks before. Turn around and put the other sock on your other foot in the same way.

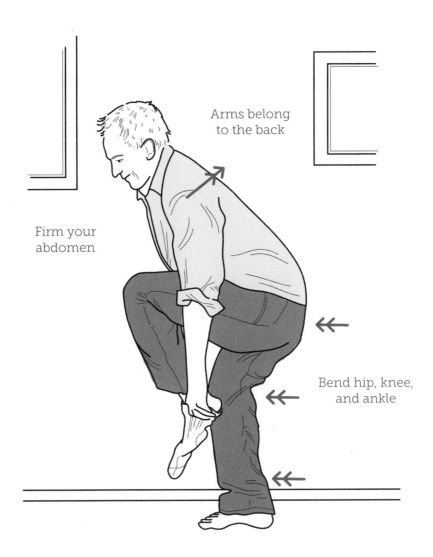

Arms belong
to the back

Firm your
abdomen

Bend hip, knee,
and ankle

3. Phone Stance No. 2—Tightrope

When you get a phone call, stand up to engage your legs as you did in Week 3. Scissor your legs to the front and back, using floorboards or an imaginary tightrope to align your front foot directly in front of your back foot. Be sure there is something nearby to steady yourself if you start to topple.

Even though your legs are not side by side as they were in "Phone Stance No. 1—Shin Bones Press In" (page 72), use the same action you used to squeeze the imaginary balloon by pressing your right shin toward the left and your left shin toward the right.

With this activation of your legs and hips, ground yourself onto the spreading tripod of the bottom of your feet, especially through the big-toe metatarsals, into the floor. At the same time, lift yourself upward from your thighs and pelvis to bring the long front body upright on top of this narrow base. Firm your abdomen to connect your upper body to your lower body. Your hip bones face straight ahead, level with each other. Your shoulders are also level over your hips, and your cheekbones are level over your shoulders. Your toes will extend forward; your heels, backward. Maintain the shin bones pressing in to keep your balance on the tightrope!

Relax the shoulder of the arm that holds the phone to your ear. Switch the arm that holds the phone and the leg that's in front each time you talk on the phone.

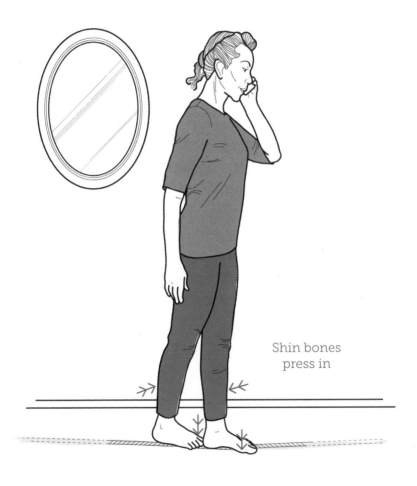

Shin bones press in

4. Checking Email Seated Upward/ Backward Bend

Whenever you find yourself sitting for a time in front of your computer, take a moment to stretch into an upward and slightly backward bend.

First, move your hips back in the chair until you feel your buttocks against the seat back. Inhale and lift your arms overhead, stretching upward from deep in the front and back of your pelvis. Open your heart high toward the ceiling while your sitting bones ground wide on the chair seat. Lean backward over the top of the seat back for support.

Don't flop your head backward. Keep your chin easily sliding toward your Adam's apple and your shoulders falling downward as your arms continue reaching upward.

Then, place your hands behind your head, elbows wide, cradling the base of your skull.

No need to hold the position. Exhale and firm your abdominals, your bottom ribs down the front toward the pelvis, while carrying your head with your hands, to return to sitting upright.

Feel the postural transformation. Breathe into your open chest.

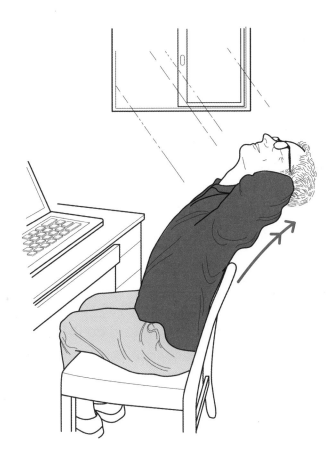

Downtime Legs up the Wall

By now you may be accustomed to using downtime at the end of the day to release tension and experience stretch. While watching TV, having a conversation, or decompressing at the day's end, sit down beside a wall and swing your legs upward as you lie down on your back. Your spine will rest neutrally on the floor and your legs will be straight up, propped high on the wall.

Don't place yourself so close to the wall that your pelvis is tilted away from the floor. Scoot away from the wall to make sure the tail end of your spine remains on the floor. Engage the muscles of the front of your thighs as though to move your legs downward into your hip sockets. Reach your heels in the opposite direction, upward on the wall. Allow the back of your neck to be long and relaxed, just like the rest of your spine. Place a slim book under your head if your neck feels constricted. Rest your arms by your sides. Breathe fully and feel the stretch sensation in the back of your legs.

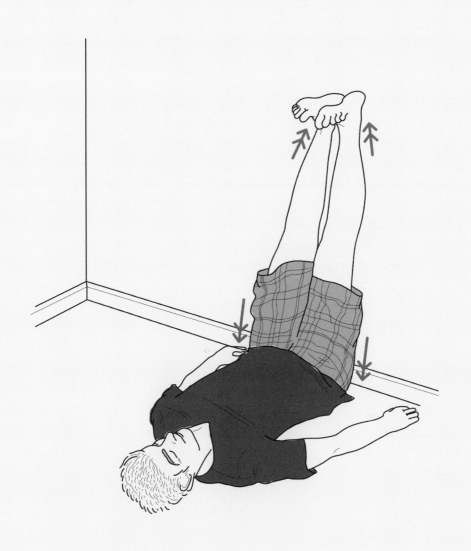

Week 7

This week, try for hands free while performing activities from the past weeks of your balance practice.

1. Step Up to Get Dressed No. 2—Not Touching Dresser

Again, place the step stool in front of your dresser. Each morning when you get dressed, do the ten step-ups on each leg, *without* touching the dresser. It's there only if you need to steady yourself.

With your right foot up on the step, bend deeply at the right ankle, which will release your knees and allow your hips to bend as well. Slowly transfer your weight from your back left leg to your right leg on the stool, contracting your buttock muscle to unbend your right hip when you step up. From the bottom of your abdomen, pull your body up on top of your right leg. Imagine your pelvis moving up and over on top of the standing leg on the step.

Pause at the top to balance on one leg before descending backward. Bend the right hip, knee, and ankle to lower yourself and transfer weight onto the left leg. Be sure to cushion the transfer by articulating your left foot and bending at the left ankle, knee, and hip. At all times, keep your right leg on the step.

Do the same on your left leg.

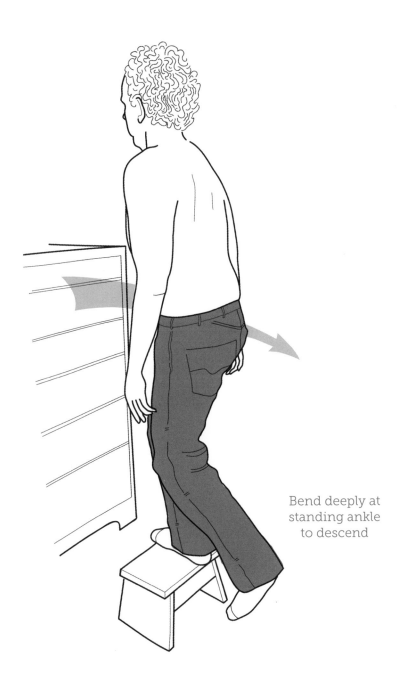

Bend deeply at
standing ankle
to descend

2. Putting on Socks No. 2— Not Touching Shoulder to Wall

Stand on one leg right next to a wall to put on each sock as in "Putting on Socks No. 1" (page 114). This time, try to do it without touching your shoulder to the wall.

Remember to allow your standing ankle, knee, and hip to release and bend as you spread your foot long and wide as a base of support. Take your time. If needed, briefly lean and touch your shoulder to the wall for stability and then slowly return to balancing without the wall's support.

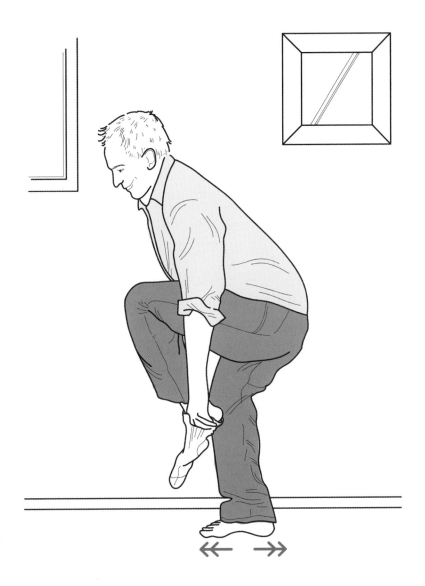

3. Forward and Backward Heel-to-Toe Tightrope Walking

Slow down as you approach your passageway (the one you used for "Walking Backward" in Week 5, page 106). This week, put one foot in front of the other as if you were walking on a tightrope. Use the floorboards for the tightrope, or put removable tape down so you will be reminded to walk the line. Your front leg's heel steps directly in front of your back leg's toes.

Keep pressing your shins in to draw your legs underneath you on the tightrope just as you did in "Phone Stance No. 2—Tightrope" (page 116.) Your right shin presses toward the left and your left shin presses toward the right. Articulate your feet with a heel-ball-toe action as you step. Drop your weight into the floor and breathe while you walk. Use your arms wide at waist level for balance.

Don't get frustrated. Losing balance and falling off the tightrope is good! Your balance system is working to right you and will improve with practice. The more you tightrope walk down the passageway, the better you will get.

If you feel confident about walking forward, the next time, walk backward on the tightrope. Articulate your feet with a toe-ball-heel action as you step backward.

If you start to waiver, relax your ankles, knees, and hips to bend and release any tightening or gripping of your body.

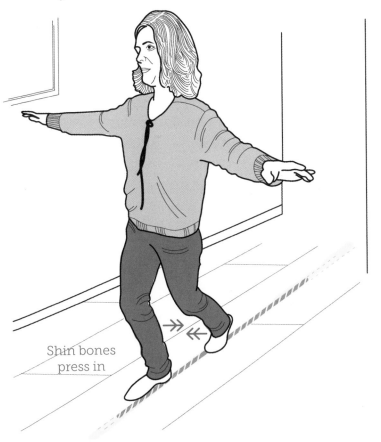

Shin bones press in

Tightrope Walking

When you are standing, a wide stance may make you feel stable, but walking with your legs far apart weakens your walking stride. Bring your feet closer together. When you are out and about this week, imagine you are walking on a tightrope, putting each foot in front of the other. You don't need to literally walk the single line of a tightrope. Simply activate your muscles as if you were.

Draw the insides of your shins toward each other, your right shin to the left and your left shin to the right—as tightrope walkers do. This activation comes upward from the inside arches of your feet, shins, and thighs along the same route as the inseam of tight jeans, and will add power to your stride.

After you get the feeling of "tightrope walking" while you walk, add it to the other cues: "helium balloon," "shoulder swagger," and "big toe push off/falling forward."

4. Sit-to-Stand Squat No. 3—Hover and Heel Lift

Use every time you sit down or stand up as a further opportunity to practice and strengthen your squat.

Cross your arms over your chest as in "Sit-to-Stand Squat No. 2" (page 90). When you are in the process of squatting down, stop when your sitting bones are very near the seat of the chair and hover there for ten seconds.

During the hover, lift you right heel so that your weight is primarily on your left leg. Keep your hips even. Put your right heel back down and ground it. Stay in the squat and lift your left heel so that your weight is squatting primarily on your right leg. Put your left heel back down and ground it. During two-legged squats, you may be favoring the stronger leg and increasing its power while the weaker leg gets weaker. Lifting the heel of one leg forces the opposite leg and hip to do all the work and to have a turn to function without help.

During the one-legged hover, maintain the lift of your pelvis from the bottom of your abdomen and by contracting your buttocks. Keep your spine relaxed and growing both upward into your skull and, in the opposite direction, downward out your tailbone.

After the hover and heel lifts, continue your descent to squat all the way down to sit on your sitting bones. Perform the same hover with heel lifts next time you squat up to standing.

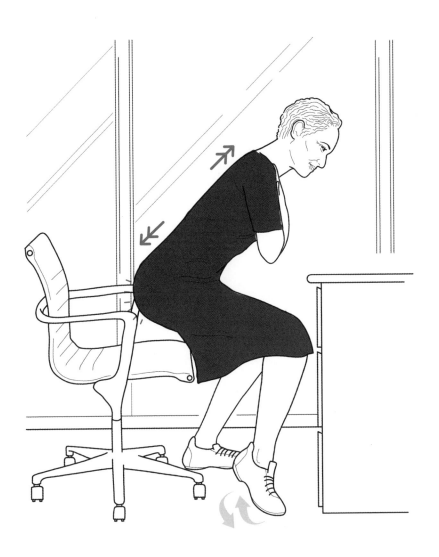

Bedtime Hanging Leg off Front Body Stretch

By now you are in the habit of doing a final stretch at the end of the day before you get in bed.

Sit down on the edge of the bed. Pull your knees up as you lower yourself backward and onto your back with both knees toward your chest. Hug them for a moment to stretch your back.

Extend your left leg off the edge of the bed so that it hangs down while you continue to hug your right knee. Breathe and relax. Feel a stretch in front of your left thigh, hip, and lower abdomen. Don't push for the stretch. Receive it passively.

Start over with both knees to your chest to extend your right leg down this time, continuing to hug your left knee, and stretch the right side of your front body.

Take at least ten slow breaths on each side. Hug both knees afterward.

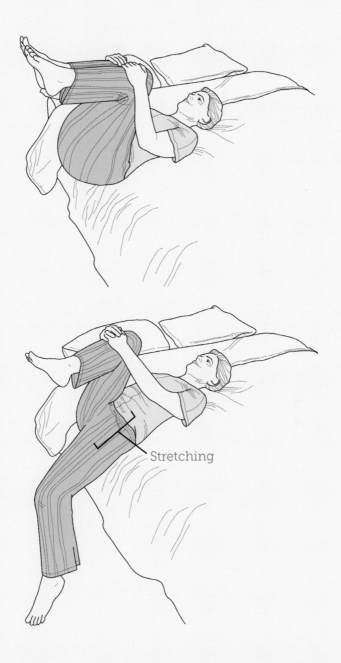

Stretching

Week 8

Good morning stretch, more strengthening, and even more challenging balancing. Step sideways for a change! Add agility to the mix this week.

Morning Stretch Backward Bend

Why not reward yourself first thing in the morning? Think of this as the classic morning stretch often depicted as a yawning, sleep-filled reach of one's arms overhead.

Keep a large bath towel near your bed so it's there in the morning when you wake up. Roll the towel into a cylinder and place it horizontally on the bed. Scoot down on your bed and lie back over the rolled towel so it's under your shoulder blades.

Reach your arms overhead in a yawning stretch and take hold of your hands if you can. If not, take hold of each elbow to rest your forearms on your forehead. Because the towel lifts your upper chest from behind, you will be arching your upper back.

Relax your lower back and hips. Support your head with a pillow if the back of your neck feels compressed.

Breathe deeply from the bottom of your belly, filling all the way up to expand your collarbones.

Repeat at least five complete breaths before you lower your arms and roll off the towel.

This is similar to "Checking Email Seated Upward/Backward Bend" (page 118) that you did in a chair during Week 6. It's another opportunity to extend your upper spine and is the remedy for stooped shoulders.

You may have an unconscious habit of blocking the intake of air that can fill upward as high as your collarbones. This inhibits the natural extension of the upper spine that accompanies the filling of the lungs in that area. Use your breath to cure your rounded upper back.

Inhale deeply to fill with air all the way up to your collarbones

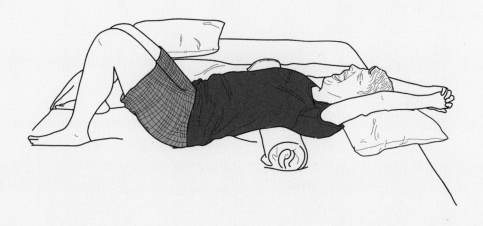

1. Putting on Socks and Pants— One Eye Closed

Each day, stand near the wall and put on your socks and pants while balancing on one leg. Alternate the leg that inserts first.

If you feel confident, try closing one eye. Touch your shoulder or hip lightly to the wall if closing one eye makes you feel too unstable. Engage your shoulder blades so that your arms belong to your back—not to your chest.

Dress Up Your Balancing Practice: Explore possibilities. Put on your socks and pants with *both* eyes closed. Stand beside the wall so you can touch your shoulder against it for stability, if needed. For a change, open your eyes and button your shirt standing on one leg. Put on tights, earrings, or gloves while balancing on one leg. Alternate legs. Take as long as you need to progress and make practicing balancing part of getting dressed every day.

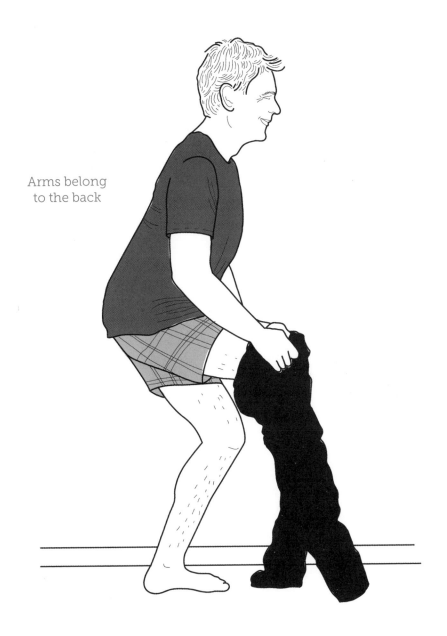

Arms belong
to the back

2. Hand Towel Sidestep Move

This one requires a bit more coordination—it is important for being agile *and* balanced.

After washing your hands or working at the kitchen sink, dry your hands and then hold the dish towel horizontally with both arms wide, stretching the towel in front of you, at waist level, between your two hands. Stand on both feet, hips-width apart.

Shift to the right, transferring your weight to the right leg as you reach your straight left leg directly to the side (not high, just barely off the ground) and bring the stretched towel upward overhead. Balance on your right leg for a second (A). The knee and toes of your left leg will be facing straight ahead, not to the ceiling.

Transfer your weight to the left onto both feet again, while bringing the stretched towel down in front of your waist back where you started (B).

Now, shift your weight to the left leg as you reach your straight right leg directly to the side and bring the towel upward overhead again. Balance on your left leg for a second (C).

Alternate stepping sideways, straight-legged, from your right to your left leg and back again, moving the outstretched towel overhead when you are on one leg and bringing the towel down when you are on both legs. Stabilize your standing hip with its buttock muscle each time you step sideways into the balance while the opposite buttock lifts the reaching leg to the side.

Alternate ten times every time you dry your hands.

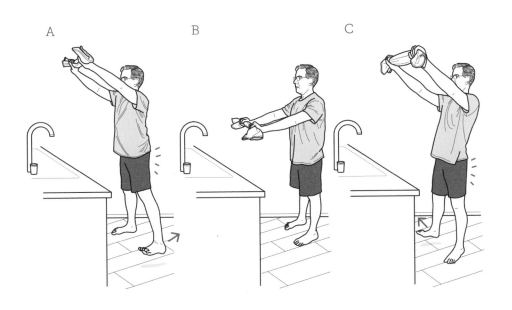

A   B   C

Repeat from side to side going through center
position B each time

3. Plank at Window Ledge No. 1

Choose a windowsill, bench, or other low sturdy furniture that you pass often. Each time you walk by, stop and place your hands on the ledge with your body at the top of a push-up position. Hold the position without doing push-ups.

Spread your fingers ahead and press downward through the knuckles of your index fingers. Turn your inner arms forward so that your elbows point behind you as they straighten. Broaden your chest. Use opposing forces to draw your arms into the sides of your back at the same time as you push your arms forward.

Create a long line of connection in your body from head to feet, like a wooden plank. You will need to firm your abdominals in the front so your rib cage and hips don't sag forward. Firm your buttocks to keep your hips straight and also firm the front of your thighs to keep your knees straight. Be careful not to bend at the hips. From the floor up, the diagonal line of your body extends like an arrow, all the way from your feet, legs, hips, and spine into your skull. Maintain the plank position for five deep breaths, increasing the number of breaths as the week goes on.

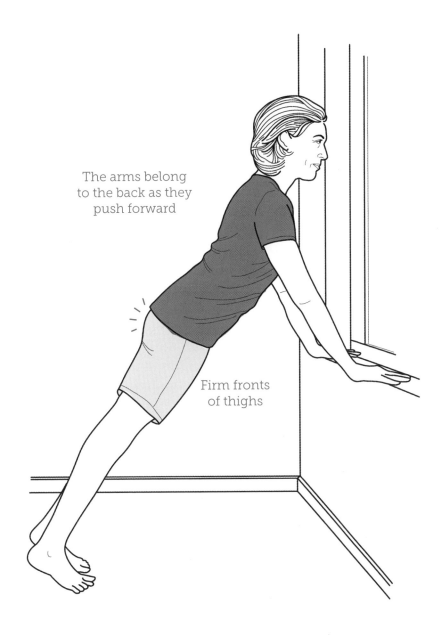

The arms belong
to the back as they
push forward

Firm fronts
of thighs

4. Grapevine Step

Here's a new move for the passageway where you've been tightrope walking. This week, whenever you take that route, walk sideways in a grapevine step.

Face away at a 90-degree angle from the direction you will travel. Step directly to the right with your right foot. Continue to travel sideways by crossing your left foot behind and placing it down slightly to the right of your right foot. Step to the right again, using your right foot. Then, step again to the right with your left foot, this time crossing it in front of your right foot. Continue the alternating pattern of stepping side-back, side-front walking.

Try it in the reverse direction when you return down the passageway, starting on the other foot. Be patient if you can't coordinate smoothly at first. With practice, over the week you will gain agility and balance.

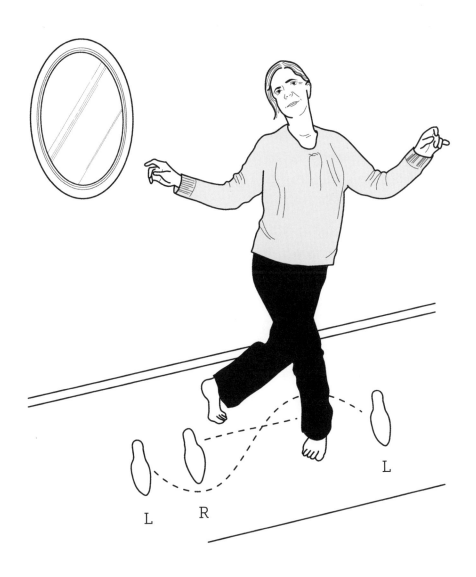

L R L

Pelvic Launch

During the past seven weeks, you've been cued to use your abdominals in the front and your buttocks in the back. It's time to work it into your walking stride.

Use butt power to walk! When you found the secret of youth in a long front body, you practiced contracting your buttock muscles to propel yourself forward into each walking step. Your buttock is responsible for launching the pelvis up and over the forward leg as you walk. Each step is pushing the earth behind you *from your hips*. Walking is less about lifting your front leg forward and more about propelling your pelvis, and entire body, from behind.

The abdominal connection unites your torso throughout the launch. Imagine raising your pelvis up from beneath your belly while your front lower ribs relax downward. Add your buttock muscles, launching your pelvis, and, with help from your big toe push-off, create the force that makes you fall forward from one foot to the other.

"Pelvic launch" is the fifth and last cue for Your Walking Stride. Practice launching your pelvis before you add it to the other four cues.

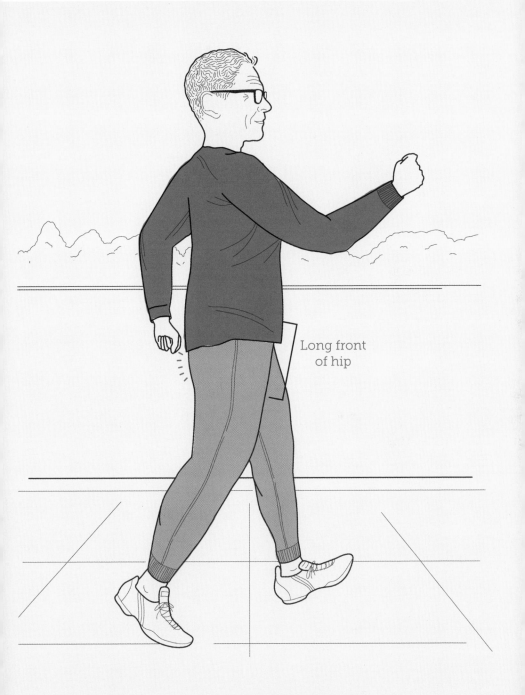

Long front
of hip

Week 9

Do you feel better about your coordination and stability when you go out and about? Continue to build more skills and confidence. Lots of stepping sideways this week!

1. Step Up Sideways to Get Dressed

Keep the step stool in front of your dresser, so that getting dressed is associated with doing the "Step Up Sideways to Get Dressed" activity.

This week, stand beside the step stool instead of facing it. Put your right foot up on the step directly beside your left foot on the ground. Place a light touch of your hands on the dresser for balance. Keep the right foot on the step at all times.

Bend your legs at the ankles, knees, and hips. When you step up and transfer your weight to your right leg, you will travel sideways. Pause briefly on top of the step on your straight right leg before you bend the right leg's ankle, knee, and hip to descend sideways, transferring weight back onto your left foot on the ground. Be sure to cushion your landing by allowing your left leg to bend at the ankle, knee and hip.

If you feel confident toward the end of the week, let go of your hands on the dresser. Stay close to the dresser as you face it, so your hands can easily stabilize you with a touch. Never stabilize with a hand placed behind you.

Step up sideways ten times, landing in a slight squat as you step down sideways.

Stand on the opposite side of the step stool with your left foot on the step and right leg on the floor. Step up sideways ten times.

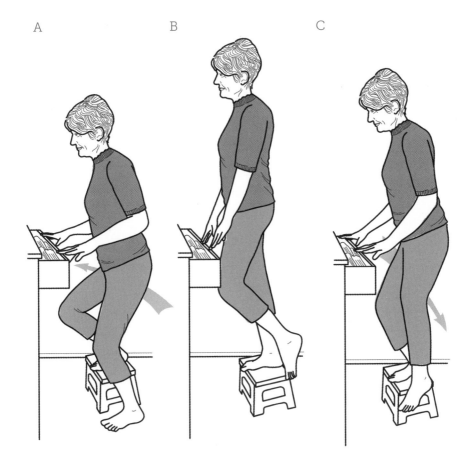

A   B   C

Habit Alert

Make toweling dry after your shower or bath a habitual opportunity for daily balance practice. It will only take a moment. After you get out of the shower or bathtub, stand safely on a bathroom rug, with a wall or sturdy surface next to you, to dry off with a towel.

Pick up your right foot and dry it while you stand on your left leg. Keep standing on your left leg while you continue toweling off your entire right leg, starting with your foot.

Step to the side to change legs. Pick up your left foot and dry the left leg, starting with the foot and toweling up the leg.

Dry off the rest of your body.

You transfer your weight sideways, stabilizing your one-legged balance act with your standing hip. You're also transferring weight sideways in "Step Up Sideways to Get Dressed" this week.

Mastering lateral moves of this kind is key to preventing falls. If you can move in only one direction (forward), how will you keep from faltering when the unexpected backward or sideways move takes you off balance?

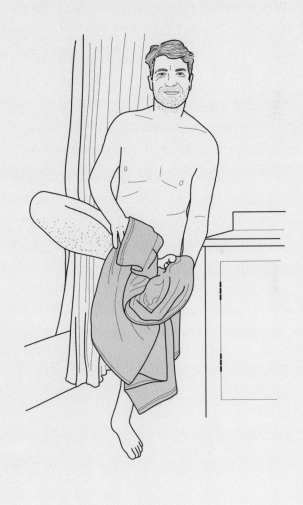

2. Body Builder's Multiple Squats

Now that you are accustomed to utilizing every opportunity of sitting down or standing up to strengthen your lower body, add eight to twelve "Sit-to-Stand Squats" using your arms for counterbalance. As you squat down your arms swing forward at waist level. As you squat up your arms fall down by your sides.

Don't sit all the way down during the squat repetitions. Lower your body until your sitting bones lightly graze the chair seat. Keep contracting your buttocks to lift your pelvis back up onto your standing legs throughout all repetitions. Think of using the bottom of your abdomen and buttocks—your core—to bring your body up on top of your legs.

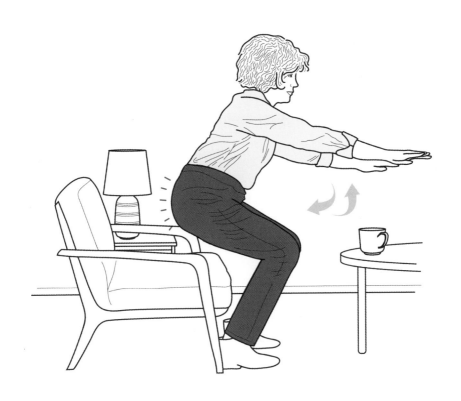

3. Plank at Window Ledge No. 2—One Leg Lifted

As in "Plank at Window Ledge No. 1" (page 144), set yourself up in the plank position when you pass the designated spot.

This week, breathe ten deep breaths while you maintain the plank position with one leg lifted off the floor.

Keep both hips in line and maintain the stability of a long wooden plank—standing on one leg this time. Keep in mind that this is not push-ups; your arms remain straight. While you breathe steadily, use opposing forces to keep the pose dynamic: Use your arms and chest to push yourself back over your standing leg; oppose that force by using the foot of your standing leg to push yourself forward. Send your entire front body toward your back body. Reach the one leg long off the ground to pull you straighter.

Alternate the leg that reaches off the ground each time you pass the ledge and take plank position.

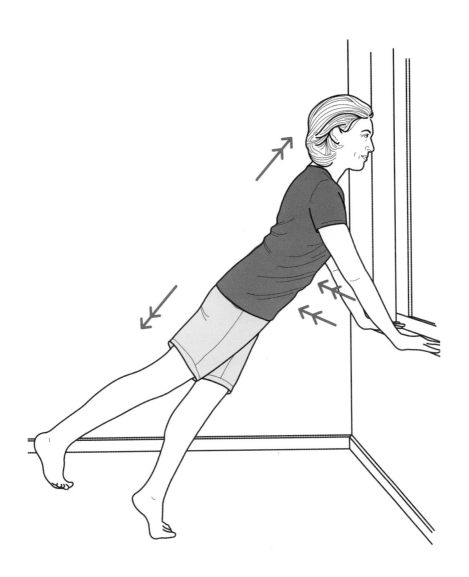

4. Slow-Motion Walking

That passageway will never be the same for you. It prompts you to challenge your coordination and balance.

During Week 9, very slowly take one step forward, lift the back leg, and pause before stepping forward again. Continue as if you're in a slow-motion film. Very, very slowly! The slower you walk, the more balance is required. Bend your ankles, knees, and hips to drop your weight.

For an even greater challenge, try it backward. Beforehand, know how many steps you can take within the space available. But don't stop there. As you become more comfortable, add another enormous challenge: Walk forward and backward at slow-motion speed with both eyes closed. Try walking backward in a circle with your eyes closed. Trust the placement of your feet on the floor and your body's position in space without visual feedback.

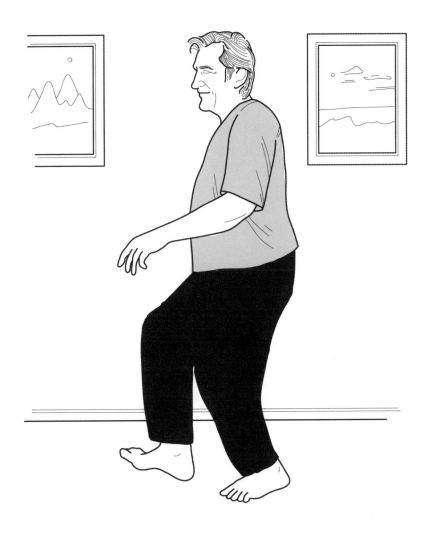

S-l-o-w-l-y

Dance to Music!

Move some furniture and put on music that makes you want to move.

Start by transferring weight from one foot to the other in time with the music. Then, begin to isolate body parts and move your head, neck, shoulders, back, rib cage, and hips. Make up your own steps or imitate moves you've seen. Test your balance with holds and accents.

Without pushing too hard, make it feel good, like stretching to get the kinks out.

Experiment with small and detailed moves, or try bigger gestures that use your greatest range of motion with control. Or lose control! But keep it safely in your own capacity. By now, you know your own body, balance, and strength. Dance to trust it.

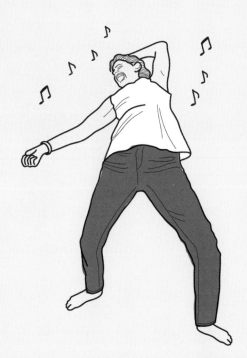

Week 10

This is your victory week! Show off your stuff.

1. Brushing Teeth Balance No. 6—Slow-Motion Marching

With your twice-daily brushing of teeth, you have plenty of opportunities to try some fancy balance work. Try slow-motion marching during morning and night brushing. *Really* slow motion. It can be a challenge to coordinate such a slow pace with your lower body while you brush your teeth at a quicker pace. You will very slowly transfer from standing on one leg with the other leg bent to the front at a 90-degree angle, your thigh and knee at hip level, and then back to the other leg, as you march in slow motion.

If you lose your balance, either lightly touch your free hand to the counter or touch one toe down to the floor until you feel stable again.

Brush Up Your Balancing Practice: Here's an optional goal: When you feel ready, slowly close both eyes while brushing and balancing on one leg. By excluding sight, you can develop your body's use of other sensory input that contributes to balancing.

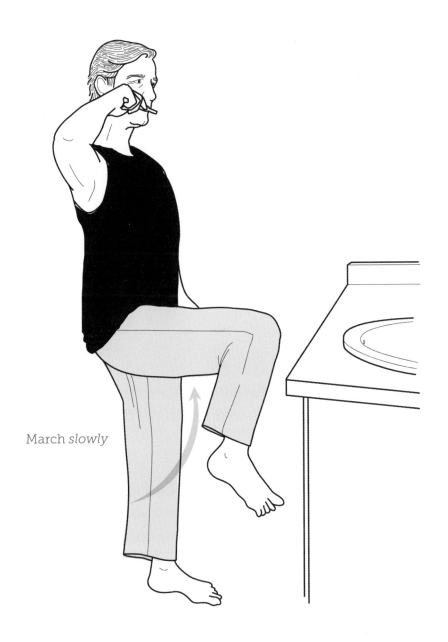

March *slowly*

2. Backward Step Up to Get Dressed

Over the past weeks, while getting dressed, you've stepped up moving forward and stepped up moving sideways. This week, you will transfer your weight backward. You may feel disoriented, just as you might have when you walked backward in Week 5. Keep your fingers lightly touching the dresser.

Stand facing the dresser with the step stool directly behind you. Your weight should be on your left foot on the floor in front of the step stool. Place your right foot behind you on the step.

Bend at both ankles, knees, and hips. To step up backward, transfer your weight onto your right leg on the step and release your left foot from the ground. Straighten your right leg to pause in the balance before bending both ankles, knees, and hips to step forward and return your weight to your left foot on the ground. At all times, keep the right foot on the step.

Remember to bend at the standing ankle, knee, and hip to prepare for the ascent and descent and to cushion the landing.

Keep your hands forward on the dresser for as many days as you need to, then try it with your arms down by your side.

If it's too difficult to manage stepping up backward, remove the step stool and step backward onto level ground. It's a great balance challenge to step backward into standing on one leg.

Every time you get dressed, perform the backward step up ten times for each leg.

A B C

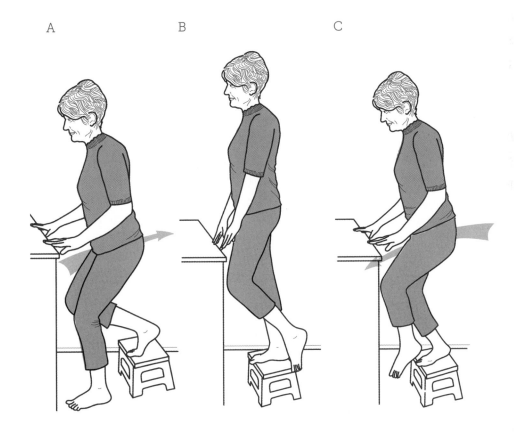

3. Window Ledge Push-ups

When you pass the designated ledge or sturdy arm of a couch, stop and align your body in the plank position.

Bend your elbows behind you to lower all the way to the ledge so that you feel your chest touching it. Push your body back up to straight arm plank position.

Avoid reaching your head down to get closer to touching the ledge with your chest. Instead, keep your head in line with the rest of your spine.

Contract your abdominals toward your spine so your ribs and hips don't sag forward. Contract your buttocks to keep your hips in line with your legs and ribs. Keep your shoulders down and away from your ears. Use your chest muscles to push up while you draw your arms and shoulder blades into the sides of your back. Broaden your chest.

Even if you only do one push-up, do it through the entire range of motion. You can increase the number of push-ups gradually. It will take many weeks to build up the number of repetitions. Don't strain. Do one or two push-ups with good form instead of more with less-than-good form.

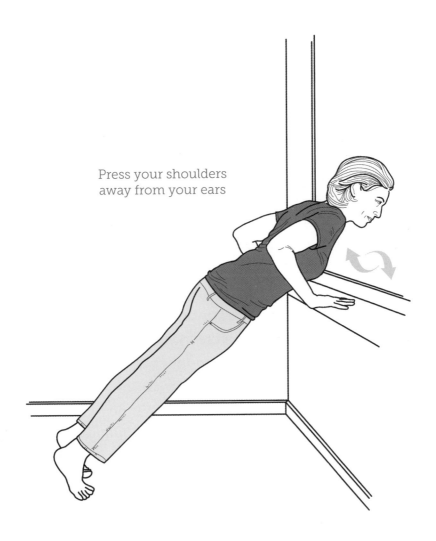

Press your shoulders
away from your ears

4. Commercial Break Split Squat with Chair

When a commercial comes on television, hop up off that couch and perform some split squats.

Face the back of a chair so that you have a light touch on the seat back. Place your right foot forward in front of your right hip and under the chair. Place the forefoot of your left foot behind your left hip, allowing your left heel to come off the ground. Your weight will be primarily on your right leg.

Squat down, allowing your hips to hinge back. Use your abdominal muscles to keep your hips lifted and squared to the chair. Use your right buttock muscle to lift your pelvis back up to starting position.

Split squat eight times and then change to the left foot in front for eight split squats on the left side. Now your weight will be primarily on your left leg throughout the squats.

Relax your shoulders down and keep them squared, like your hips. Don't let the front knee bend farther forward than your front toes.

Afterward, when the commercial is over, sit down in the chair and do "Seated Groin Stretch" and "Seated Back of Thigh Stretch."

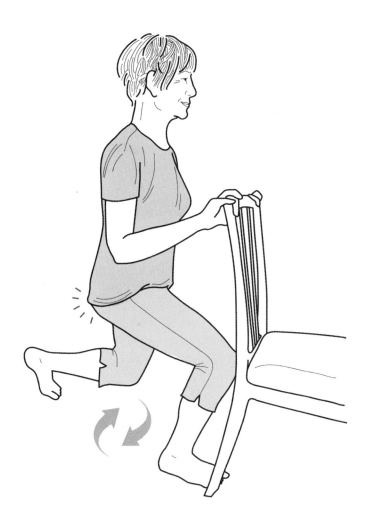

Seated Groin Stretch: Sit sideways in the chair facing left so that your left foot is forward, knee bent at a 90-degree angle, and your right leg is back behind you with the knee dipping down. You are straddling the chair seat facing sideways. Bring your pelvis upright and activate your abdominal muscles so that your pubic bone is zipping up to your navel like the zipper of the fly of your pants. Feel the stretch in front of your right hip and groin while you breathe for a minute. Turn the opposite direction and stretch the front of the left hip.

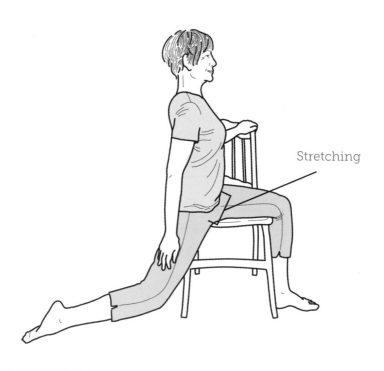

Stretching

Seated Back of Thigh Stretch: Sit facing the correct way in the chair with your right leg extended straight out in front and your left leg bent under the chair. Lean forward at the hip with a flat back. Slide your right hip backward on the seat of the chair and direct your right heel forward. Feel the muscle of the front of your right thigh contracting and feel the muscle of the back of your right thigh stretching. Don't force your back or hunch into tilting forward. Bend where the thigh bone meets your pelvis and keep your spine extended. Change legs to stretch the back of the left thigh.

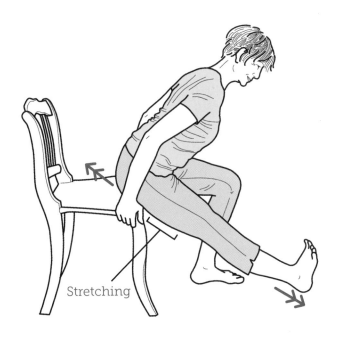

Stretching

Combine All Five Cues

Go for a walk. Put all five cues together from the top down: "helium balloon," "shoulder swagger," "pelvic launch," "tightrope walking," and "big toe push off/falling forward." Walking well is unifying your body's posture and mechanics for power and function. If you combine all the cues, walking will make you stronger instead of wearing you out!

Your balance will improve as a result of the strength and connections you use in your walking stride.

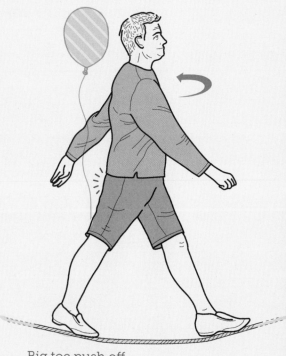

Big toe push off

Moving On

Neurological Balance Exercises

Give it a shot. You will find it interesting to perform these tricks. Integrate eye and head movement and stimulate your brain's balance control system.

1. "Yes" and "No" Exercise

Stand on one leg with the other leg hovering just above the floor. Focus on an object a good distance in front of you. Slowly nod your head as if to say yes for a while. Keep breathing and keep your eyes focused on the visual target.

Slowly shake your head as if to say no for a while. Keep your eyes fixed on the target object.

Change to standing on the other leg and repeat. Make it easier by standing on two legs with your feet together.

2. Walking "Yes" and "No" Exercise

Find a good distance to walk in your home so you can walk forward keeping your eyes fixed on a target ahead. Nod yes while you walk, stopping when you almost reach the target object.

Walk backward to the starting point, and then walk forward, again, shaking your head no. Visual focus is key.

For a further challenge, you can try both the "yes" and "no" nods while walking backward, as well.

3. Eyes Fixed/Eyes Moving Rotational Balance Exercise

Stand on one leg. Hold your arms straight out in front of your chest with the palms together.

Keep your eyes fixed straight ahead on a visual target while you turn your torso above the waist to the right and then to the left ten times. Your eyes should not turn to follow the rotation of your torso. Your head and arms will rotate with your torso. Stand on the other leg and repeat.

Now do the same exercise, but instead of focusing on a single object, allow your eyes to move in the same direction as your head and arms when you rotate. Your vision will simultaneously follow the direction in which you rotate. You will see everything along the way instead of focusing on one target.

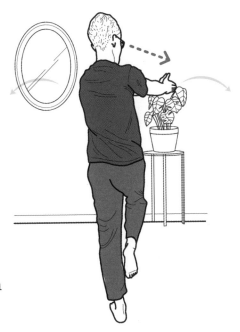

Which visual instruction makes it harder to balance, fixed eyes or moving eyes?

Make the exercise easier to perform by standing on both legs with your feet together.

What If You Do Fall?

Even with all your improved balance and agility, accidents can happen. Coming out of a restaurant, you may be distracted while talking to someone and not see a step down. Or you might slip on a banana peel!

Nonstop Spiraling

The instant you realize you're going to fall, intercept your first reaction of fear and tension. Instead, relax and soften. Think "spiral downward." This will naturally set in motion a sequence of events: You will pivot and shift your weight, bend your joints, and present the meatier sides of your thighs, hips, back, or shoulders for consecutive contact with the ground. Stiffening with forward or backward falling would encourage catching yourself with extended arms and outreached hands. The rigidity in your arms and neck puts your wrists, elbows, and head at risk for injury. You don't want to hit bony end points, such as your tailbone or kneecap, either. With spiraling, you go with the momentum of the fall—rounding, tucking, and spreading the impact on the way.

Let's practice no-hands spiraling. Stand close beside a wall on your right-hand side.

Begin by rotating your upper body to the right and loosening your legs to descend partway down, pivoting on your feet and leaning toward the wall until your left buttock touches the wall for support. You will have made a half-turn.

Don't touch the wall with your hands at any time during the spiral. Relax as you turn and trust that you will gently contact the wall with your hip.

Reverse the spiral, facing the opposite direction.

Now practice spiraling all the way to the floor, without the wall for support at the halfway point. Stand on a surface with some give, such as a thick rug. Rotate your body as before, while bending your legs at the ankles, knees, and hips, rounding your spine and allowing your head to bow forward slightly. Instead of using your arms and hands to make contact with the floor, commit to continual bending and revolving in your legs and body. The key is to never stop pivoting and spiraling. If you hesitate and stop turning, if only for a split second, you will hit heavily. Aim to continue the spiral during and *after* the contact. Your fleshy hips, sides of your back, or shoulders will move continuously through contact with the floor. I repeat. Never stop the turning motion. Keep rolling on the floor until the momentum and force is completely used up and you are lying on the ground quietly.

As another releasing and coordination exercise, try reversing the spiraling sequence from the floor back up to standing. For daily practice, stand and spiral all the way down to the floor and back up again. Change the direction of the spiral each time to use a different side of your body's strength and flexibility.

All this spiraling practice will put you at decreased risk for breaking bones and straining muscles, if or when you do fall.

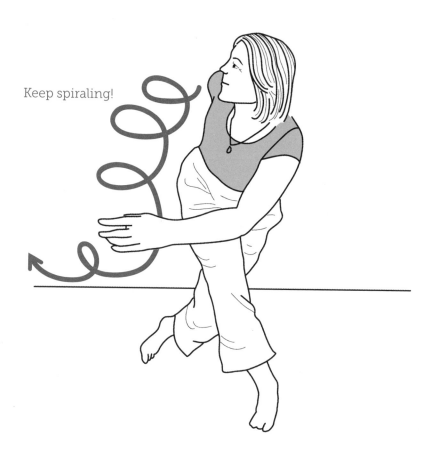

Keep spiraling!

If You Fall

After a fall, stay calm and still. Before you try to stand up, consider whether you are injured. You want to prevent falling down again while getting back up or, worse, falling immediately after you've recaptured the standing upright position.

The Pep Talk

Stuart was diagnosed with peripheral neuropathy. He went around to all the best doctors and physical therapists, demanding that this numbness and weakness from damaged nerves in his feet would not continue to deteriorate his balance. But he was constantly battling falling. They said there was nothing to be done.

Stuart began to put on his favorite dance music and allow his body to move itself in ways that were rhythmic and pleasurable, moves that offered stretching and swaying, reaching, kicking, changing direction, and snapping fingers. After a few months, he had made up a dance that he could repeat daily. He's still dancing into his nineties. He calls it his balance routine.

The human body was designed to move.

OK, this is the game plan. Don't give up; keep moving. The temptation to give in to the sitting disease may be great. You may yearn to slow down. If you aren't naturally inspired and motivated to keep physically active, then you may have to encourage yourself, force yourself, meet with a partner, do whatever it takes to make it easier or acceptable or mandatory—to move. Try everything. Keep looking for physical activities that sustain you in the moment, and that are fun. Have you tried croquet? Billiards? Tai Chi? Baton twirling? Ping-pong? Contra dancing, gardening, kite flying, bird watching, or joining a marching band? Just about any activity done while standing up will improve your balance.

The more you move, the better your balance. The better your balance, the greater your confidence. Don't give up hope. Keep trying.

Acknowledgments

I appreciate the patient help of Batya Rosenblum at The Experiment. I am grateful to Jon LaPook for going the extra mile for me. Sincere thanks to my friend Joseph Hannan, for his good-natured advice on the manuscript. To those who put in some overtime coming to my aid: Chistopher Berg, Natalie Houchins, Henry Murdock, Julie Waugh, and Livia Whitermore. And thank you, Kate Gyllenhaal, a pioneer in the field of personal training, and Dr. George Russell, the bodyworker of all bodywork. Honor is due to Susan Halseth and her clavicle at JM CLASS. I am in awe of the encouragement, support, service, and generosity of spirit of my once-in-a-lifetime mate, Richard Murdock. You actually believe in me. Finally, I thank the miraculously positive and clever Joan Strasbaugh, also a believer, without whom this book would not exist.

About the Author

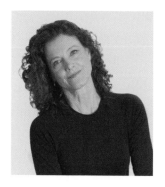

With a background in dance and choreography, Carol Clements is a teacher of many movement arts, techniques, and methods. She works with her private clients in New York City.